PILATES
FOR LIFE

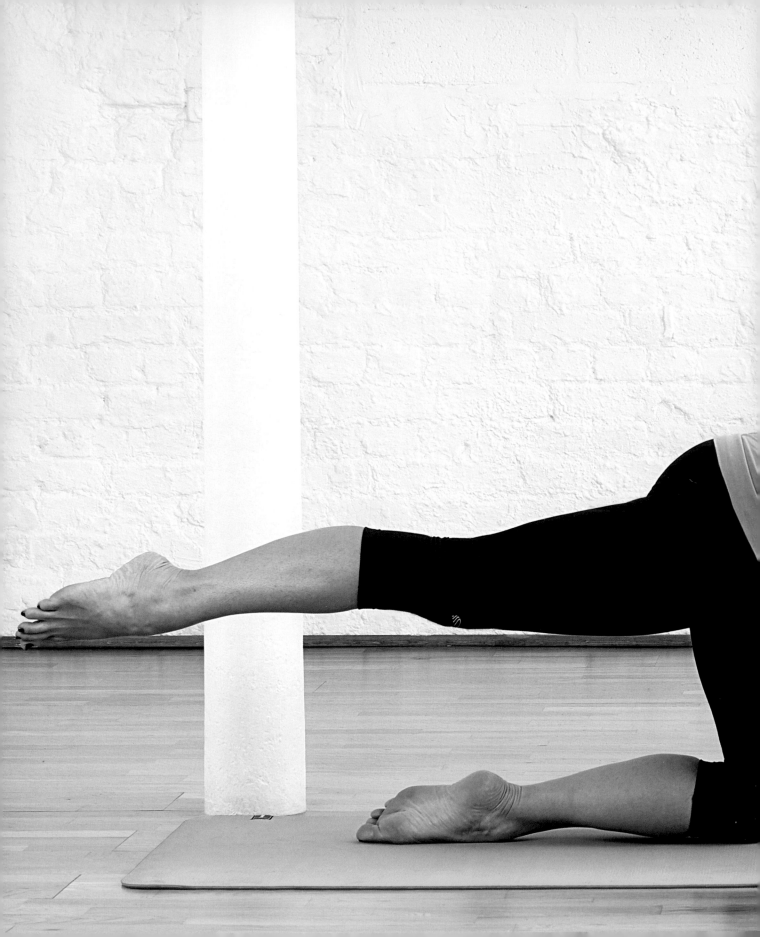

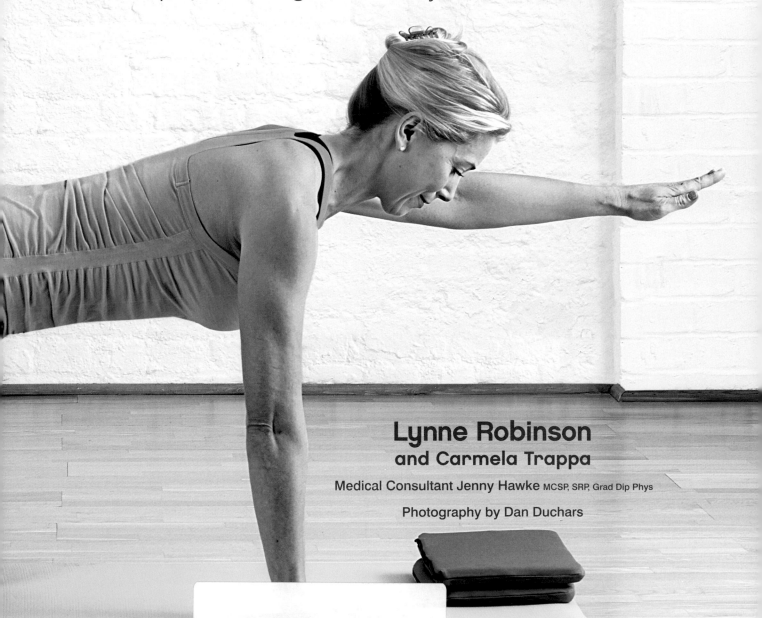

PILATES FOR LIFE

How to improve strength, flexibility and health over 40

Lynne Robinson
and Carmela Trappa

Medical Consultant Jenny Hawke MCSP, SRP, Grad Dip Phys

Photography by Dan Duchars

Kyle Books

For our families

First published in Great Britain in 2014 by
Kyle Books, an imprint of Kyle Cathie Ltd
192–198 Vauxhall Bridge Road
London SW1V 1DX
general.enquiries@kylebooks.com
www.kylebooks.com

Printer line 10 9 8 7 6 5 4 3 2

ISBN 978 0 85783 218 4

Editors: Catharine Robertson and Tara O'Sullivan
Copy Editor: Anne Newman
Designer: Jenny Semple
Photographer: Dan Duchars
Production: Lisa Pinnell

A Cataloguing in Publication record for this title is available from the British Library.

Colour reproduction by ALTA London
Printed and bound in China by C & C Offset Printing Co.

Disclaimer: The author and publisher cannot accept any responsibility for misadventure resulting from the practice of any of the techniques or principles in this book. It is not intended to be and should not be used as guidance for the treatment of serious health problems; please refer to a medical professional if you have concerns about any aspect of your condition or fitness level.

CONTENTS

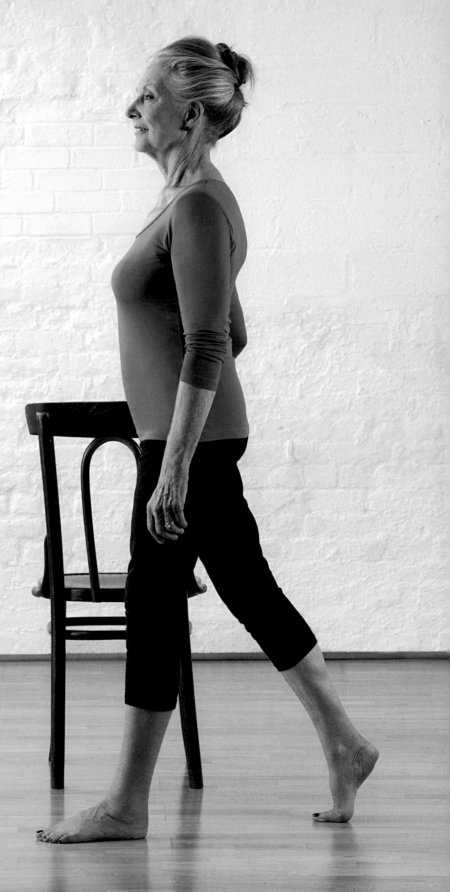

INTRODUCTION

We now have the opportunity to live longer than we have at any time in history. Over the last 150 years there has been a dramatic increase in life expectancy in developed countries, with the figure rising by two and a half years per decade. This means that a quarter of all babies that were born in 2013 have the potential to live to be 100 years old.

So we have the chance to enjoy our life for longer, but how can we ensure that we will be fit and healthy enough to enjoy the extra years? The answer is very simple, and has been known for centuries. Roger Bacon, the 13th-century Franciscan friar, wrote a book on ageing in which he proposed that the effects of old age could be postponed by eating a controlled diet, getting proper rest and plenty of exercise, and practising good hygiene and moderation in all aspects of our lifestyle. And although today there is a mountain of research on successful ageing – or ageing well – so far (at the time of going to press) no one has come up with a magic pill, and Roger Bacon's message is still clear: use it or lose it.

Most of the changes attributed to ageing are actually caused in large part by disuse. So adopting as healthy and active a lifestyle as possible is the best health insurance there is. We may not be able to stop the ageing process completely, but we have it within our control to slow down the clock! In fact, research shows that the normal ageing process can be delayed by 10 to 20 years by participating in regular physical activity (Shepard 1997).

So whether you are 40 or 80, it is never too early – or late – to start looking after your mind and your body. We should strive to maintain a dynamic balance between mind–body wellbeing and social interaction and relationships in order to enjoy successful and harmonious ageing.

'Physical activity is one of the most effective ways of positively influencing our health. Regular exercise can lower our risk of getting serious conditions, such as stroke, heart disease and certain cancers. It can add years to our lives, but most importantly, it keeps us happy and helps us maintain our independence.'

Age UK

In this book we are going to introduce you to the ultimate anti-ageing Pilates exercise programme, specially designed not only to keep you active, but also to help you glow with vitality and good health. It is no coincidence that, for decades, celebrities have used Pilates to keep their minds and bodies youthful. Sian Phillips who, at 80 years of age, is still performing on stage and screen across the globe, says: 'Regular Pilates sessions, regardless of mood, weather or inclination, are the only way I can maintain my fitness and enjoy life.'

This method works!

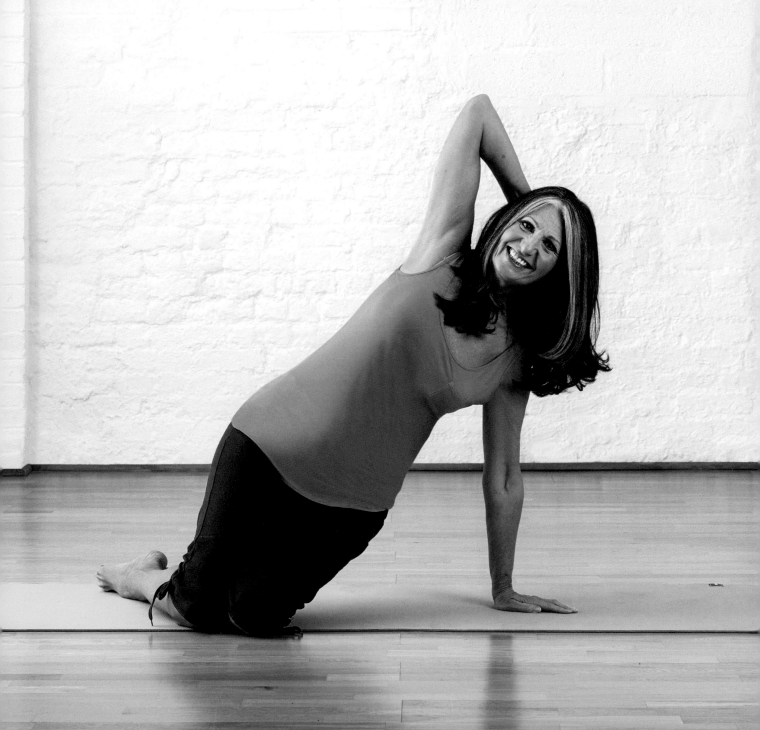

'And exercise thy lasting youth defends.'

English poet John Gay (1685–1732)

WHO IS THIS BOOK FOR AND WHAT ARE THE BENEFITS?

We have aimed this book at everyone over the age of 40. Why 40? Because this is the age when, if you have not already started, you will need to start investing in your future health. You will read later in the book that this is the age at which your bones start to lose density and muscles weaken. It is also the age when you need to be more selective about which exercises are going to help you the most. And we refuse to put an upper age limit on the programme – whether you are 40 or 90, a Pilates veteran or a novice, super-fit or not, you will find this programme invaluable.

Pilates is for life and can be life-changing. It is not only a form of exercise – it also offers a different way of understanding the body and how it moves. Pilates does require a level of commitment to bring about changes, but as it is so rewarding, many people are happy to make that commitment. This is why Pilates is enjoying popularity worldwide.

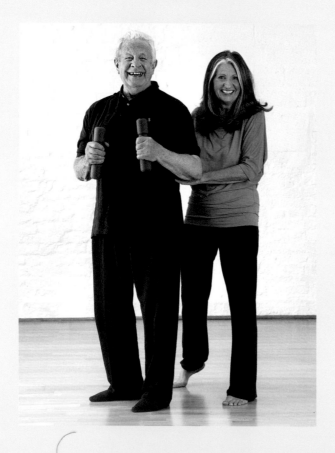

And the benefits? The changes experienced by people who do regular Pilates can include any of the following:

■ increased flexibility and strength of the spine
■ increased mobility (range of movement) in all major joints and management of joint conditions
■ improved posture
■ improved balance and associated reduced risk of falls
■ improved co-ordination
■ more efficient breathing and management of respiratory conditions
■ improved bone strength
■ increased stamina and energy
■ stronger muscles – in particular the gluteals, quadriceps, hamstrings, calves, upper arm, back and, of course, the abdominal and pelvic-floor muscles
■ a more streamlined outline, in particular a trimmer waistline
■ improved dexterity and grip
■ healthier, less painful feet
■ a lessening of pain in some health conditions
■ improved sleep patterns
■ improved self-esteem and confidence
■ less stress
■ improved ability to carry out daily activities
■ help with maintaining independence
■ help in managing conditions of the mind and emotions
■ a feeling of general health and wellbeing.

That is quite a list! Remember, too, that Pilates is both mind- and body-conditioning. As Joseph Pilates writes in his book *Your Health*: it is 'NOT MIND OR BODY BUT MIND AND BODY [his capitals]... man should develop his physical condition simultaneously with the development of his mind – neither should be sacrificed at the expense of the other.' The body shapes the way we think, and thinking influences the body. By learning new exercises and new movement patterns you can train the brain alongside the body. Pilates requires you to move with precision, which means you have to constantly be aware of what you are doing and attain excellence through practice.

Throughout our lives we move in certain ways and, over the years, habits can develop which affect our normal movement patterns. Each time we move to do something, certain muscles are switched on by our brains in a particular order which, when we are young, is an efficient and natural way to move. However, as the years progress, our movements change, which can then lead to some muscles weakening. In response, other muscles compensate for this 'imbalance' by trying to do the job of the weakened muscle. This then sets up a movement pattern which is not efficient and can lead to poor alignment, causing an increased likelihood of wear and tear, and ultimately pain. Pilates offers an incredibly safe way to exercise and to realign the body and change the way you move.

Pilates can give you the awareness, strength and flexibility to stand tall regardless of your age – so the classic stooped posture we associate with ageing need not be inevitable. However, we must recognise that for successful ageing, Pilates alone is not enough. You will need to look after your heart and include some cardiovascular activities, which is why we have included a section on heart health (pp.172–74). You will also need to follow a healthy, balanced diet.

We are very aware that most adults over the age of 65 may be living with one or more chronic medical conditions, such as osteoarthritis, osteoporosis or Parkinson's. With this in mind, you will find exercise programmes designed specifically to help with the management of conditions commonly associated with ageing (pp.146–216). We are determined to keep you active!

'If I'd known I was going to live this long, I would have taken better care of myself.'

Attributed to ragtime composer Eubie Blake, who lived to 100.

THE LEGACY OF JOSEPH PILATES (1883–1967)

If you are going to follow a particular exercise method, it is always reassuring to know that its creator lived a long and healthy life. In fact, exactly how old Joseph Pilates was is a matter of controversy. We know he died in 1967 in Lenox Hill Hospital, New York. And he always gave his birth date as 1880. However, on investigation, the birth registry in his birthplace (Mönchengladbach, Germany) shows his birth date as 1883. Whichever date is correct, to live to around 80 at a time when the average life expectancy was so much lower is testament to his resilience; especially given that he had suffered as a child from asthma, rickets and rheumatic fever. He survived against the odds and held the firm conviction that we each have to take responsibility for our own health.

The link between happiness, health and fitness became Pilates's passion. Elements of other disciplines – including yoga, martial arts, gymnastics, skiing, self-defence, dance, circus training and weight training – can be recognised in Joe's later teaching. By absorbing and selecting the most effective aspects from each, he was able to develop a system which had the perfect balance of strength and flexibility.

In the 1920s, Joe and his wife Clara set up the first 'Contrology' studio on Eighth Avenue in New York. While the first studio clients were predominantly male – many from the boxing community – the nearby New York City Ballet encouraged its dancers to seek Joe out when they were injured. Many of these went on to become his assistants and greatly influenced the way in which his method evolved. The original exercises that Joe created were mat-based but, over time, in order to help build strength and flexibility and to supplement those matwork exercises, he created various pieces of studio equipment.

'Joseph was a passionate, larger-than-life figure who ran the studio with a rod of iron.'

Joe wrote two books – *Return to Life Through Contrology* (1945) and *Your Health* (1934). In them, he expressed his concern for the health of most Americans. He felt that it was only through regular practice of his exercises that people would 'return to life'. It was in his studio that the Pilates Method as we know it today was defined. Joseph was a passionate, larger-than-life figure who ran the studio with a rod of iron. Loved and respected by his clients, Joe never doubted that one day his method would become popular worldwide. Just how right he was in many of his ideas on both health and fitness makes him nothing short of a visionary.

Joe exercised right up until his death. There are even reports of him wandering the corridors of Lenox Hill Hospital trying to get other patients to exercise! His first disciples (often called 'First Generation Teachers') are a testament to the benefits of Pilates: Mary Bowen is in her eighties and is, at the time of writing, still travelling, teaching and inspiring everyone she meets; Lolita San Miguel is still teaching her wonderful classes all over the world; Ron Fletcher and Romana Kryzanowska were both 90 when they died; Carola Trier was a mere youngster when she passed away in 2000, aged 87! It seems that Pilates and longevity go hand in hand.

HOW IS THIS BOOK DIFFERENT FROM OTHER PILATES BOOKS?

In order to make the Pilates for Life programme more effective against the effects of ageing, we have modified many of the traditional exercises and created exciting brand new ones. We aim to give you the strength, flexibility and motor skills you need to keep fit, active and independent for the rest of your life. The format of the programme may look unfamiliar to a regular Pilates devotee – for example, you will find many more back-extension exercises (such as the Dart) than is usual, as we are aiming to reverse the more negative effects of gravity on the body and iron out any effects of years spent at a desk by strengthening the upper-back muscles. But don't worry – we won't be ignoring those abdominal muscles! Neither will we ignore your gluteal (buttock) muscles, as these are crucial later in life and are often neglected. In fact, no part will be ignored – even the pelvic floor gets its own section!

You will find lots more standing exercises to improve your balance and help prevent falls. We have to keep your joints aligned, mobile and supported by strong muscles in perfect balance. In the section on osteoporosis (pp. 146–55)you will see we recommend far more repetitions and heavier weights than normal. This is because we need to load your bones in order to build density.

In a nutshell, we hope to both stimulate you mentally and challenge you physically into staying younger longer!

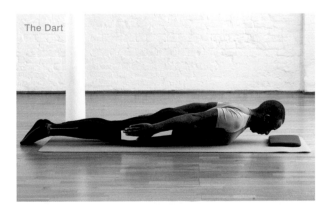

The Dart

The Body Control Pilates Approach

There are now many different schools of Pilates, each with its own approach to teaching Joe's work. The Pilates for Life programme is part of the Body Control Pilates syllabus. Founded in 1995, Body Control Pilates aimed to make the benefits of Pilates as accessible as possible to everyone, irrespective of age, income and fitness level.

We recognised that there was a demand for a more structured and modern approach to teaching the Pilates method and, with this in mind, we created a unique programme that takes you progressively and safely towards Joseph Pilates's original work.

We have always believed that it is the quality of teaching which defines good Pilates, and we are proud that Body Control Pilates is widely seen as a benchmark for safe and effective mat- and machine-teaching of the highest quality. Our education courses are now delivered in over 15 countries and our curriculum contains more than 30 different courses to help our teachers in their professional development.

Our headquarters are in Bloomsbury in the heart of London, where we operate public classes and studio teaching as well as our teacher training courses. The Body Control Pilates Association is Europe's largest professional Pilates body with more than 1,400 teaching members based in over 40 countries and it is our fervent hope that this book inspires you to hunt out a Body Control Pilates teacher near you.

www.bodycontrolpilates.com

MEASURING AGE

This is much more controversial than you would imagine. Professor Lewis Wolpert writes in his excellent book on ageing, 'old age is by no means easy to define. It is a biological phenomenon characterised by certain physical changes that take place with time and also by their psychological consequences. It is the changes in individual appearance that prompt your friends to remark, "You're looking very well",' (this being the title of his book).

The obvious way to measure age is to look at a person's birth date. But as the milestones of 40, 50, 60, 70, 80, 90 and 100 are approached and, hopefully, passed, most people will agree that these are simply numbers which give little indication of our health or how we feel.

In 1979 the Harvard psychologist Professor Ellen Langer conducted a groundbreaking experiment which demonstrated clearly just how much power the mind has over our health. Professor Langer recruited a group of men in their late 70s and 80s into what she described as retreat which would be 'a week of reminiscence'. There was no mention of ageing. Before they entered the retreat, Professor Langer measured their gait, dexterity, arthritis, speed of movement, cognitive abilities, memory, and so on.

Professor Langer then divided the men into two groups. The first group was the control group and they were encouraged to reminisce about their lives in the 1950s. The other group were secluded in a house which was full of props from the 1950s. Everything in the house – from the TV programmes and the news to the food – was from that time, and the men were asked to live as if it were 1959. To encourage them to reconnect with their younger selves, all 'elderly' aids (like stair rails) were removed from the house. They were not helped with their suitcases or treated as 'elderly' or sick in any way – quite the contrary. It was not long before these men were making their own meals and walking faster. One man decided he did not need his walking stick at all.

At the end of the week, all the men were tested again. Both groups showed improvements in their physiological measurements, with a drop in blood pressure and even improvements in hearing and eyesight. But the second group's results were noticeably better. By encouraging the men's minds to *think* younger, their bodies had followed and they had become 'younger'.

So if our birth date is an inadequate measure of our age, how else can we measure it? We can look at our 'functional' age – this relates to our levels of fitness and ability to perform daily activities. For example, a woman of 60 who does regular aerobic exercise may have the functional age of a woman of 45 with respect to aerobic fitness.

Another approach is to assess genetic and cellular damage within the body, in particular the body's ability to repair and regenerate. About 30–40 per cent of the ageing process can be attributed to genetics (Rowe and Kahn 1998). It is only a few genes which affect the rate at which we age; many more of our genes carry the potential for developing chronic conditions.

*2005 Article Weikart PS. Movement and the brain-body connection in N. A. Brickman, H. Barton & J. Burd (Eds) Supporting Young Learners 4: Ideas for child care providers and teachers Ypsilanti, MI: High Scope Press

Other theories about ageing include the activity theory, which is probably the best known social theory. This stipulates that if you stay engaged in mental or physical activities throughout your life, you are more likely to age in a healthier and happier way (Fisher 1995; Lemon, Bengston and Peterson 1972). Since our mental capacity can also decline with age, perhaps in a less obvious way than any outward physical changes, it is no less important to our happiness in older age.

In terms of how we age psychologically, seven key factors have emerged: emotional intelligence, cognitive capacity, self-efficacy (our belief in our own ability to do things independently), self-esteem, personal control, coping style and resilience.

So can Pilates have an impact on any of the above? Well, there may not be anything we can do about your chronological age, but we can certainly help you look younger, feel better about yourself, be more confident and also improve the way you move through your day. The Pilates for Life exercises have been designed specifically to be functional, to enable you to perform your everyday tasks easily.

Through Pilates you will be using your body as a learning tool. In her article on Movement and the brain–body connection* Phyllis S. Weikart pointed out that in our formative years, purposeful movement is essential to our development because intentional movements engage the brain and develop essential links between thinking, language and movement–brain–body connections. There is no reason we should stop this learning later in life! Once called 'the thinking person's exercise' (by osteopath Andrew Ferguson DO MSc), your mind is certainly engaged in Pilates as you co-ordinate your breath, control your alignment and move with precision. Pilates aims to stimulate you mentally as well as physically.

'Physical fitness is the first requisite of happiness. Our interpretation of physical fitness is the attainment and maintenance of a uniformly developed body with a sound mind fully capable of naturally, easily and satisfactorily performing our many and varied daily tasks with spontaneous zest and pleasure.'

Return to Life Through Contrology, Joseph Pilates

THE PROCESS OF AGEING

Ageing is a natural part of the life cycle. It is not an illness.

Cells, muscles and bones

Although we have aimed this programme at those aged 40-plus, change is happening at a cellular level within our bodies from the point of conception until we die.

All our cells change as we age, becoming less efficient. This affects the connective tissue within our joints, making them increasingly stiff and less mobile. Tendons which connect muscles to bone, and ligaments which connect bone to bone, become less elastic and tear more easily. There is a decrease in production of the synovial fluid which is essential for lubricating our joints. Wear and tear may result in cartilage and bone degeneration. Less flexibility is probably one of the first things we notice, alongside the wrinkles and the greying hair! However, not everyone is affected in the same way. The more active you are, the more flexible you will be, especially around the hips, spine, ankles and knees (Daly and Spinks 2000). This is why increasing joint mobility will be high on our list of exercise priorities.

Ageing affects all our body's systems, but not all at the same rate. In addition to the normal changes associated with ageing there are age-related conditions. The main causes of physiological decline are chronic (long-term) conditions affecting our cardiovascular, metabolic, musculoskeletal and neurological systems. A decline in one of these systems has a knock-on effect and may increase our fragility or cause further disability.

'If your spine is inflexibly stiff at 30, you are old; if it is completely flexible at 60, you are young.'

Return to Life Through Contrology, Joseph Pilates

Our muscles lose strength as we grow older, with both the amount and size of muscle fibres decreasing. Muscle mass decreases by about 20 per cent between the ages of 20 and 70, with some studies suggesting that the average body loses around 3kg of lean muscle every decade from middle age onwards. This may sound depressing, but much depends on the amount of physical activity we do throughout our lives – and remember, it is never too late to start.

It is not just our muscles which may weaken – our bones do too. We start to lose bone density from about the age of 35, though the rate of calcium loss in women during the five years following the menopause (Drinkwater 1994) makes women three times more likely to develop osteoporosis than men. On pp. 146–47 we will be exploring in greater depth the effects of exercise on bone density.

As well as bones becoming more fragile, our intervertebral discs are also affected by ageing. These discs of cartilage play a crucial role in acting as shock absorbers for our spines. As we age, these discs shrink and hold less water, so we can feel a shortening in the spine and experience some changes in posture, although we have much more control over our posture than we imagine. Poor posture is never inherited. Elongation of the spine is one of our primary goals in the programme, alongside teaching you to articulate the spine, thus keeping it flexible.

Heart

As we have seen, some of the changes associated with ageing start much earlier than you would imagine. After age 25–30, for example, the average man's maximum attainable heart rate declines by about one beat per minute, per year, and his heart's peak capacity to pump blood drifts down by 5–10 per cent per decade. In everyday terms, the diminished aerobic capacity can produce fatigue and breathlessness with modest daily activities. Although Pilates is not an aerobic style of exercise, we have included some valuable advice on cardiovascular activities on pp. 172–73.

'By the time you're 80 years old, you've learned everything. You only have to remember it.' George Burns

Breathing

Ageing affects our respiratory system, too, as our lung capacity decreases. As one of our guiding principles, learning to breathe in a better way is fundamental to Pilates and is one of the first things you will learn in this programme

Joseph Pilates was convinced of the role of breathing well in promoting longevity. In *Return to Life Through Contrology* he wrote: 'Breathing is the first act of life and the last. Our very life depends on it. Since we cannot live without breathing it is tragically deplorable to contemplate the millions and millions who have never learned to master the art of correct breathing. One often wonders how so many millions continue to live as long as they do under this tremendous handicap to longevity.'

Memory

And then there's the impact of ageing on our minds. Memory has been shown to decline from around the age of 40. As we age, our brain shrinks due to fluid and cell reduction. And as the number of nerve cells decreases, our reflexes become slower as peripheral nerves conduct impulses more slowly. This also results in decreased sensation. We need longer to process information and find it increasingly difficult to multitask. We have dedicated a special section to mental health, where we will consider the benefits of exercise for stress, depression and dementia.

Eyesight and hearing

How many of you are reading this book with the help of reading glasses? Both vision and hearing decline with age. The combined changes to our cognitive, sensory and motor systems affect our stability, balance and co-ordination.

If the above processes sound rather depressing, do please note that we are all individuals and we will all age differently and at different rates. There are some aspects of ageing over which we have very little control. Thankfully, however, there are many more about which we can and will make a difference. As we have said, we may not be able to stop the clock ticking, but we will do our best to slow it down.
You have already taken the first step by purchasing this book. Next, you need to find out how to use it.

HOW TO USE THIS BOOK

Everything you need to know for good Pilates practice is contained within this book. But where do you start?

Regardless of your Pilates experience, we would recommend that you start with The Fundamentals (pp. 20-83), which covers all the basic movement skills of our approach and forms the foundation on which the whole programme is built. Even if you have years of Pilates experience, you should still find this chapter informative and extremely useful. Under each of the headings 'Alignment', 'Breathing' and 'Centring', there are exercises which help to illustrate these fundamental skills. At the start of each exercise, we explain its primary focus and provide a note of caution if you have a particular medical condition. If you are in any doubt at all, please check with your medical practitioner. Then read each exercise through several times before attempting to do it.

Always take time to find the correct Starting Alignment as this will impact the precision of your movements; you will find the different Starting Positions, such as Relaxation Position and Four-point Kneeling, in the Alignment section on pp. 22–35. Make sure that you fully understand all the movements described in the Action points. The photographs will give you a visual image of what you are trying to achieve. The Watchpoints, marked by a large asterisk, will give you tips on how to perfect your technique and avoid common pitfalls.

We have a built a natural progression through the programme which will allow you to work at your own pace and build your skills step by step. This is one of the strengths of the Body Control Pilates approach.

Once you have worked through The Fundamentals, you can move on to the Pilates for Life Main Exercise Programme, which is suitable for most people. This is followed by a special chapter on common health problems, Pilates for Health (pp. 144–216), offering advice on how to exercise safely with specific medical conditions and outlining exercises which are particularly beneficial. This advice must be used in conjunction with any medical guidance you have been given. You can then try the special workouts. Eventually, you will be able to plan your own workouts, but you will find some suggested workouts on pp. 82–83 and pp. 142–43.

Ideally, we would like you to aim for three hours of practice per week, but don't worry if this is not possible; even a little Pilates practice – providing it is done regularly – will make a huge difference. And, importantly, whatever you learn in Pilates should not be limited to your Pilates sessions, but should be integrated into your daily life. We have planned this programme to be as relevant as possible to maintaining the strength and flexibility needed for your everyday activities, but you need to remain aware of your posture and how you are using your body. In other words – take your Pilates with you wherever you go!

BEFORE YOU BEGIN

Here is a list of the equipment you will need for the programmes.

- A padded non-slip mat
- A folded towel or small, flat pillow
- A bed pillow
- A stretch band of medium strength or a long, stretchy scarf
- A sturdy chair
- A clear stretch of wall space
- Ankle weights *
- Hand-held weights *
- A tennis ball or equivalent

* How heavy will depend on which exercise you are doing and how good your technique is.

Your exercise space

Always prepare the space in which you are going to exercise by making it warm, comfortable and free from distractions. Make sure that you have enough room to move your arms and legs without knocking any ornaments or bumping into coffee tables. If you like, you can play some background music, but it should be quiet and not off-putting. You might also find a mirror helpful initially, so you can check your alignment.

Clothing

Wear clothing that allows for freedom of movement, but that also allows you to check your alignment. Barefoot is best, but you may also wear non-slip socks. If you know that you are unsteady on your feet, you may wear light, flexible-soled shoes for the standing exercises.

Approach

When you finish an exercise, always return, mindfully, to the Starting Position. The number of repetitions given is the ideal number for you to work towards, but not at the expense of quality of movement.

To help you learn an exercise, we have given you 'right' and 'left' instructions. When you are ready to include the exercise in your workouts, alternate the side/direction you start with each time you work out. This will help to ensure balance.

Never rush into or out of an exercise. If you are unsteady on your feet then use the method pictured on the right to get down on to your mat (unless you have your own strategy for getting down safely.) You may need a sturdy chair by your mat, or you could position your mat by a sturdy wall.

When you have finished the exercises, roll on to your side before reversing the method to get up safely. Never leap up.

Contraindications

Please do not exercise if:
■ you are feeling unwell
■ you have just eaten a heavy meal
■ you have been drinking alcohol
■ you are in pain from injury
■ you have been taking strong painkillers
■ you are undergoing medical treatment or are taking medication

Remember, it is always wise to consult your doctor/medical practitioner before taking up a new exercise regime. If you have a medical condition this is essential.

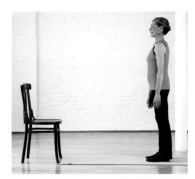
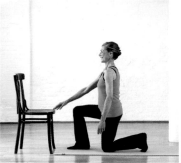
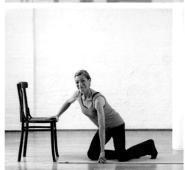
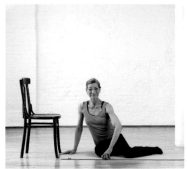
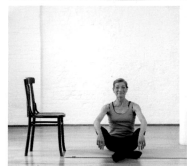

THE EIGHT GUIDING PRINCIPLES OF BODY CONTROL PILATES

The Body Control Pilates approach is underpinned by the Eight Principles of:

- Concentration
- Relaxation
- Alignment
- Breathing
- Centring
- Co-ordination
- Flowing movements
- Stamina.

Concentration

The Pilates Method was developed as both mind and body training. In order to bring about change to the way you move, the body and mind need to work together. Joseph Pilates taught that one of the main results of his method is gaining the mastery of your mind over the complete control of your body. He drew inspiration from the martial arts – slow, controlled, flowing movements performed with thoughtful awareness. Good Pilates practice requires precision of movement which, in turn, requires you to be 'present' and mindful of your whole body while you exercise. Think of it as movement meditation. This patterning of your movements is one of our primary goals. Regular practice and repetition of the movements mean that they become muscle memories, but this does not mean you can switch off. One of the joys of Pilates is that there is always another level of refinement, another challenge and new depths of understanding of the work to explore.

Relaxation

It may seem contradictory for relaxation to be a principle of an exercise method, but relaxation of the mind and body is an essential part of any Pilates session. Focusing on releasing areas of tension within the body before, and during, each exercise is important as it allows constructive change to occur. As you focus completely on your movements, your mind feels clearer and free from stress. If you hold on to unnecessary tension, the overactive muscles that tend to dominate your movements will continue to do so. This is the rationale behind taking a few moments at the start of your session to 'tune in' to your body, to allow any areas of tension to release. The Relaxation Position is ideal for this. As you become more proficient you will be able to use any of the Starting Positions or even one of your favourite preparation exercises to achieve the same thing. Spine Curls is a popular choice at the start of a workout.

Alignment

The first of the Fundamental Principles which we will be exploring in greater depth (pp. 22–35), correct alignment at the start and throughout the movement, is absolutely essential. By correctly aligning the body and controlling the position of your joints you encourage sound movement patterns, efficient breathing and stability. It also ensures there is no undue stress on your joints. Good posture and precision of movement are key to good Pilates practice.

Breathing

Breathing is our second Fundamental Principle (pp. 36–37). Breath is the essence of life itself. It is a movement process in its own right and therefore has great bearing on the efficiency of each movement the body performs. The muscles involved in the breathing process are also crucial to postural control. Synchronising the breath to movements is a key part of Pilates. With any movement in Pilates, we are looking for precision and efficiency, and breathing is no different; learning how to breathe more effectively within movement helps both the mind and body to relax, recharge and focus.

'Learning how to breathe more effectively within movement helps both the mind and body to relax.'

Centring

Our third Fundamental Principle, Centring (pp. 38–53), is probably the one Pilates is most famous for, but it is also the most misunderstood. It has come to mean so many different things to different people, both within and outside the Pilates community; depending on your school of Pilates, Centring is also often referred to as 'core stability' or 'using the powerhouse'. It encourages the deep core muscles to help control and stabilise the movement process. Centring, however, is a dynamic process that relates directly to both the challenge of limiting any unwanted movement, as well as maintaining the control and flow of the movements that are supposed to be taking place at any given moment throughout the exercise. All Pilates movements stem from a strong centre. The recruitment of the muscles involved in the centring process should reflect the demands of the movement being performed.

Co-ordination

There is no doubt that some of us are born with better co-ordination than others! But practice will improve your co-ordination skills. The programme we have developed in this book will help your co-ordination skills gradually, step by step, and will also help to maintain them by challenging you with increasingly difficult combinations of movement. Each movement, whether simple or complex, should be performed purposefully, with precision and control.

Flowing movements

Pilates exercises should always be performed with fluidity and grace – flowing movements, controlled and lengthening outwards from a strong centre. Occasionally, you may be asked to hold a position in a Pilates exercise (this will be to develop endurance and stamina, another of our guiding principles), but the majority of Pilates exercises are dynamic and should flow. This is one of the major differences between Pilates and yoga. You will learn how to control the articulation of your spine through flexion, extension, side flexion and rotation, to move the spine bone by bone. Similarly, you will be mobilising your joints, taking them through their normal ranges of movement. The end result is healthier joints. Your muscles will be longer and stronger as they are taken through their entire range. This, in turn, promotes a more efficient movement system across the whole body.

Stamina (muscular endurance)

You will be amazed at how regular practice of Pilates will increase your stamina. Even though each exercise is performed for relatively few repetitions, when part of a balanced workout each will work in harmony with the others to gradually build endurance into your muscles. As your movements and breathing become more efficient, and good posture becomes natural to you, you will find you have much more energy. Treat the recommended number of repetitions as a guideline only; stop when you feel the quality of your movements is compromised, but do work towards the suggested number of repetitions, so that your muscles become stronger. As you make progress, be sure to add more challenging exercises; keep moving your goalposts.

THE FUNDAMENTALS

While the Eight Principles outlined on pages 18–19 underpin our whole approach, three of them form the Fundamentals of Pilates – the basics which need to be mastered before you attempt any of the exercises and which deserve to be revisited on a regular basis to reinforce good practice. They will be the foundation of all your training.

These Fundamentals can conveniently be labelled as the 'ABCs of Pilates' – Alignment, Breathing and Centring – and must be tackled in the right order. So it is crucial that you consider your alignment before you think about your breathing, and both your alignment and your breathing before you think about connecting to your core. In fact, by controlling your alignment and breathing, you will be controlling your core!

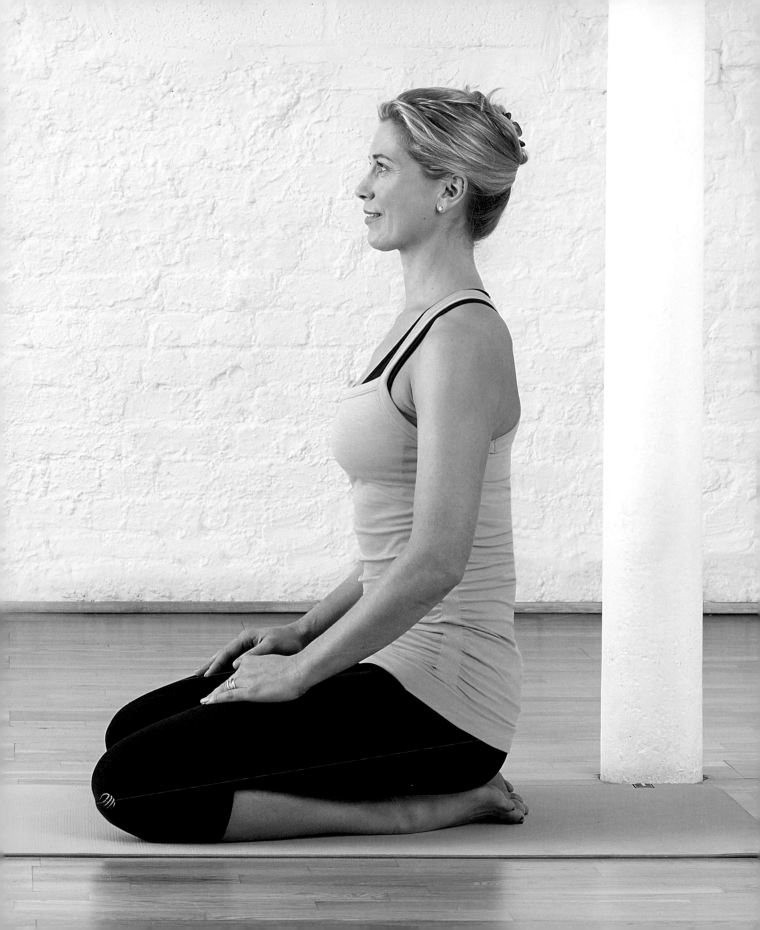

ALIGNMENT

Poor postural alignment 'switches off' your core stabilising muscles. Slouching inhibits your deep abdominal muscle, the transversus abdominis, and your pelvic-floor muscles, as well as preventing your main breathing muscle – the diaphragm – from descending properly as you breathe in. Conversely, sitting and standing tall enables all these muscles to function correctly.

We have already discussed the importance of finding good alignment before you start an exercise and maintaining it throughout. You should also be aware of returning back to the Starting Position at the end of each exercise. Awareness of where your body is in space and of where your joints are is called proprioception. Good proprioceptive skills are one of the main benefits of regular practice. In an ideal world, you would have a well-qualified teacher helping you to find perfect alignment; however when you are working alone from a book it is even more vital to get your Starting Positions correct and to follow the directions precisely. A well-placed mirror is very helpful to this end. It also enables you to check you are lying central on your mat. In the absence of a mirror, you can always use floorboards, skirting boards or walls as reference points to double-check that you are lying straight – but beware of old buildings, where these things are often not straight at all!

You will also need to learn how to recognise when your spine has maintained its natural S shape and curves. We are aiming to lengthen along the central axis of the spine in all the exercises to counter the effects of gravity over the years. There is nothing more ageing than a hunched, collapsed spine.

Similarly, you will need to know when your pelvis is in its neutral position. The Compass exercise (p. 24) will help you with this.

'The secret of joy in work is contained in one word – Excellence. To know how to do something well is to enjoy it.'

Pearl Buck

Relaxation Position

This exercise gives you the opportunity to tune into your body and organise it ready for movement. It may also be used for relaxation time, in which case you may use more pillows for support. Time spent relaxing in this position (20 minutes would be perfect) allows fluid to be reabsorbed into the discs, thus allowing the spine to release and lengthen out again. Perfect excuse for an afternoon rest!

When you are confident that you can find the Relaxation Position, move on to the Compass (p. 24). When you see Relaxation Position as a Starting Position for an exercise, you should be in your neutral position.

Starting Position

Lie on your back on a mat. Bend your knees and place the soles of your feet firmly on the mat; your legs should be hip-width apart and parallel with one another.

Lengthen and release your neck, allowing its natural curves to be maintained. If necessary, place a small, firm, flat cushion or folded towel underneath your head. The arm position varies depending on the exercise about to be performed.

Either: Place your hands on your lower abdomen with your elbows bent, resting on the mat or with a folded towel under each one (to bring them in line with your shoulders).

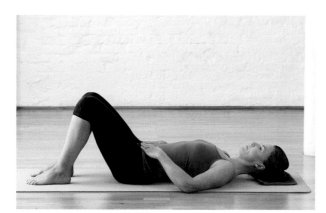

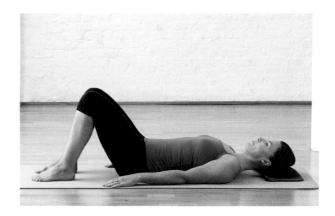

Or: Lengthen your arms by your sides on the mat with your palms facing down.

When coming out of this position, please roll on to your side and rest a moment before coming up.

■ Allow your entire spine to widen and lengthen as it relaxes and feel supported by the mat. If you use additional props for comfort when resting in this position, they will need to be removed before exercise.

■ Focus on your three areas of body weight: your ribcage, your pelvis and your head.

■ Be aware of the parts of the body that are in touch with the mat and encourage them to feel heavy and supported. In your lower spine, you will feel less contact with the mat.

■ Allow your thighs to sink down towards your hips and your lower legs towards the ankles; allow your feet to be grounded.

■ Focus on the width across your chest and feel release in the breastbone.

■ Feel lengthened in your neck and soften your jaw and forehead.

■ Allow time for the body to settle and the spine to release.

The Compass

This exercise is designed to help you develop an awareness of neutral alignment around the pelvis and lower spine. It is also a great way to mobilise and release the lower back.

* Caution: if you have a back problem or osteoporosis please take care (or avoid) going south! *

Starting Position

The Relaxation Position (p. 23), lengthening your arms by your sides on the mat. (Please note we have shown our model with her arms raised so you can see her alignment.) Now, imagine that there is a compass on your lower abdomen; your navel is north, your pubic bone is south and the prominent bones of your pelvis on either side are west and east.

Action

1 Breathe in, preparing your body to move.

2 Breathe out as you gently tilt your pelvis to the north (the pubic bone moves forwards and up). Feel your lower spine release into the mat as your pelvis tilts backwards.

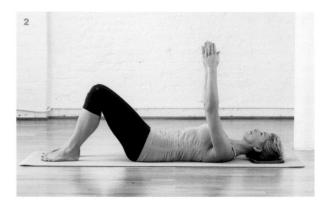

3 Breathe in as you tilt your pelvis back through the mid-position, without stopping, until the pelvis tilts gently forwards to the south (the pubic bone moves backwards and down). Your lower back will arch slightly. Repeat this north/south tilt 5 times.

4 Now, return to the Starting Position and find your neutral position, which is the mid-position – that is, neither north nor south, but in between.

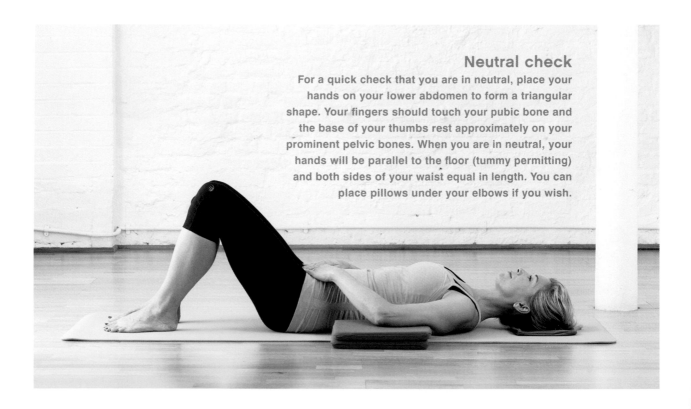

Neutral check

For a quick check that you are in neutral, place your hands on your lower abdomen to form a triangular shape. Your fingers should touch your pubic bone and the base of your thumbs rest approximately on your prominent pelvic bones. When you are in neutral, your hands will be parallel to the floor (tummy permitting) and both sides of your waist equal in length. You can place pillows under your elbows if you wish.

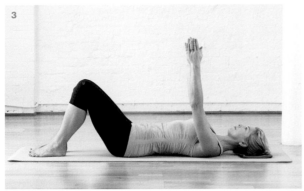

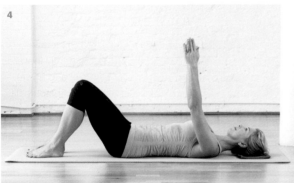

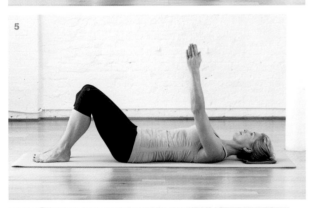

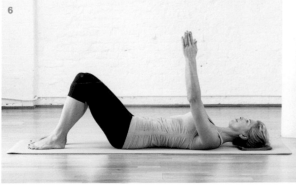

5 Breathe out as you roll your pelvis to one side – west. Feel the opposite side of the pelvis lift slightly as the pelvis rotates. Try to roll directly to the side without shortening one side of your waist (that is, without hip hiking).

6 Breathe in as you roll your pelvis through the mid-position, without stopping, to the other side – east. Feel the opposite side of your pelvis lift slightly as your pelvis rotates.

7 Return to the mid-position (neither east, west, north nor south, but in between). Your pelvis is now level. This is your neutral position.

When coming out of this position, please roll on to your side and rest a moment before coming up.

- The tilting of your pelvis should be small and achieved with ease. The rest of your spine will react slightly, but do not overexaggerate this.

- The final position of neutral should feel natural and comfortable. It must not feel fixed or rigid.

- In neutral you should feel the back of the pelvis heavy and grounded into the mat.

- Ensure that your waist is equally lengthened on both sides.

- Also ensure that there is equal weight on both sides of the pelvis.

- Allow your hip joints to be free and released.

- Once you have found neutral pelvis, do not forget about the rest of the body. Run through all of the watchpoints in Relaxation Position (p. 23).

Next we can focus more specifically on the correct alignment of the head and neck relative to the rest of the spine.

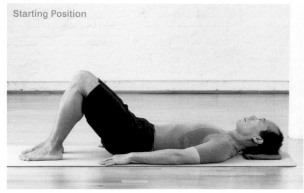

Starting Position

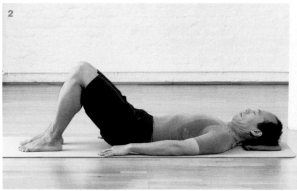

2

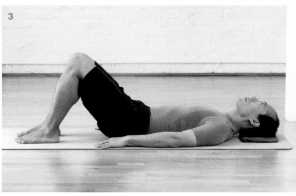

3

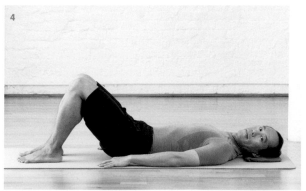

4

Chin Tucks and Neck Rolls

As we age, the bones of the neck sometimes change, due to poor posture, and wear and tear, tipping the head forwards and compressing the throat. This is a Compass-style exercise, but for the head and neck, and is designed to help you develop an awareness of neutral alignment in that area, which can be very beneficial. It is also a really effective way to release tension in the head and neck.

✻ Caution: if you have had neck, circulatory (for example a stroke) or vestibular problems, please avoid tipping the head backwards. ✻

Starting Position
Take up the Relaxation Position, lengthening your arms by your sides on the mat.

Action
1 Breathe in, preparing your body to move.

2 Breathe out as you lengthen the back of the neck and nod your head forwards, drawing the chin down. Keep your head in contact with the mat.

3 Breathe in as you tip your head back gently, passing through the mid-position without stopping, to slightly extend your neck. Once again, keep the back of the head in contact with the mat as the chin glides upwards; this is a small and subtle movement.

Repeat the Chin Tuck 5 times and then find the mid-position where your head is neither tipped back or forwards and your neck is neither flexed nor extended. This is neutral, with both your face and your focus directed towards the ceiling.

4 Breathe out as you keep your neck released, and roll your head to one side. Again, make sure that you keep your head in contact with the mat.

5 Breathe in as you roll your head back to the centre. Repeat to the other side and repeat the Neck Roll up to 5 times before returning your head back to the centre, keeping even length on both sides of your neck.

The Nod and Neck Rolls

This useful version of the Chin Tucks/Neck Rolls exercise opposite helps you identify where the 'nod' comes from and how to rotate the head and neck on a central axis.

Starting Position

Sit tall on a sturdy chair. Lightly clasp your hands behind your neck, positioning them carefully on the neck (not on the head – see the photo); in this way the neck is supported, but the head can move freely.

Action

1 Breathe in, preparing your body to move.

2 Breathe out as you lengthen the back of the neck and tip your head forwards, drawing the chin down in a nodding action. Note that the neck itself does not move.

3 Breathe in as you tip your head back gently to the start position.

4 Repeat the Nod 5 times and then release your hands and allow your head to balance freely on top of your spine.

5 Breathe in to prepare.

6 Breathe out as you slowly turn your gaze, then your head, then your neck to the right. Keep lengthening and spiralling upwards as you turn.

7 Breathe in as you slowly turn your gaze, head and neck back to the start positions, spiralling upwards as you turn.

Repeat the Neck Rolls 3 times on each side.

Variation

Try the nod with your tongue on the roof of your mouth.

* ■ Keep your jaw relaxed.

■ As you turn your head, visualise your head turning on the central axis of your spine.

■ Allow your collarbones to open as you turn.

■ Try not to disturb the natural, neutral curves of your upper and lower back.

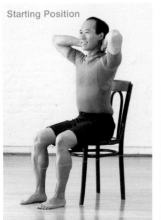

Starting Position

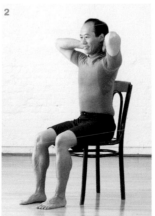

2

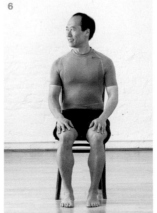

6

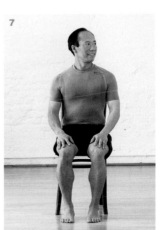

7

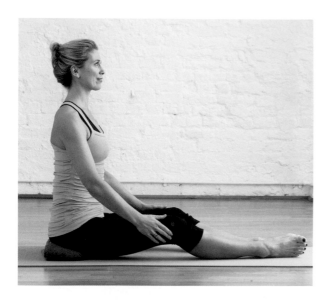

Seated Starting Positions

You will find a variety of seated Starting Positions in the book. The arm and leg positions will vary.

Seated on a Mat (Long Frog)

Sit upright on the mat. For some people it's more comfortable on a rolled-up towel or cushion as this helps you into a neutral spine position.

Bend your knees and turn your legs out from the hips and connect the soles of your feet.

Your feet should be quite a distance from the body to allow a feeling of space in the hip joints. Place your hands on the outside of your thighs/knees; your arms are lengthened, but the elbows are slightly bent.

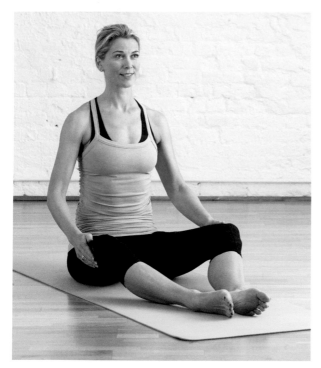

■ Ensure that your weight is balanced in the centre of your sitting bones. You should roll neither too far forwards, thereby arching your lower back, nor rock too far back, thereby flattening your lower back.

■ Lengthen your spine and be aware of the subtle, natural curvature of the lower spine.

■ Allow your ribcage to be relaxed and positioned directly above the pelvis, neither swaying backwards nor slumping forwards.

Seated on a Chair

If you are going to use a chair for exercise it needs to be a sturdy, upright one. For some exercises you will need an armless chair.

■ Sit tall on your sitting bones. You can feel these when you sit on a hard chair and place your hands under each buttock. By transferring your weight from cheek to cheek, you can feel the sitting bones. The weight should be evenly distributed between those bones.

■ Have your feet planted hip-width apart either on the floor

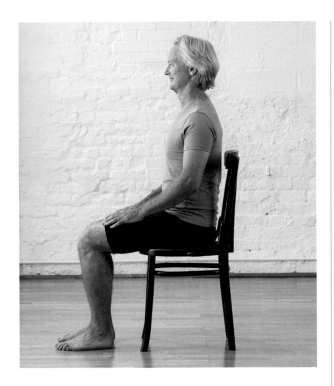

or, if you are a bit short in the leg, on a low step or pile of books.

■ There should be at least 5cm between your knee and the seat edge, so as not to restrict blood circulation to the lower leg. Keep your back long with its natural 'S curve' still present. Slouching makes a collapsed C shape and increases the pressure on joints and discs.

■ Supporting the lower (lumbar) back is sometimes necessary, especially if your core stabilising muscles are not yet strong enough to do the job. You may use a small cushion as support.

■ Lengthen your spine and allow the subtle, natural curvature of the lower spine.

■ Allow your ribcage to relax and be positioned directly above the pelvis, neither swaying backwards nor slumping forwards.

■ Relax your shoulders, feel the collarbones open and wide.

■ Allow your head to balance freely on top of your spine.

Hand Press

This simple action is incredibly useful as it can be done discreetly anytime and anywhere (as long as you are sitting down). It will help you find the axial length of your spine, that is, the position where your spine is elongated.

Starting Position

Sit on a chair as described, but place the back of each hand on the top of each thigh, fingers pointing inwards as shown.

Action

1 Breathe in to prepare to move.

2 Breathe out as you gently, but firmly, press down through the back of each hand and simultaneously lengthen up and away through your spine.

3 Breathe in and hold this lengthened position.

4 Breathe out and relax, but do not collapse.
Repeat up to 8 times.

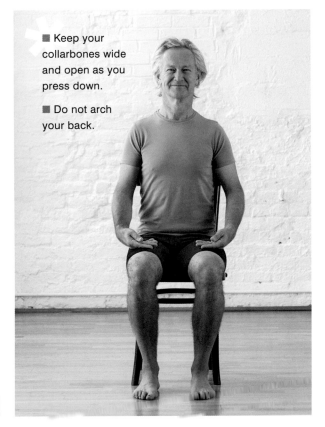

■ Keep your collarbones wide and open as you press down.

■ Do not arch your back.

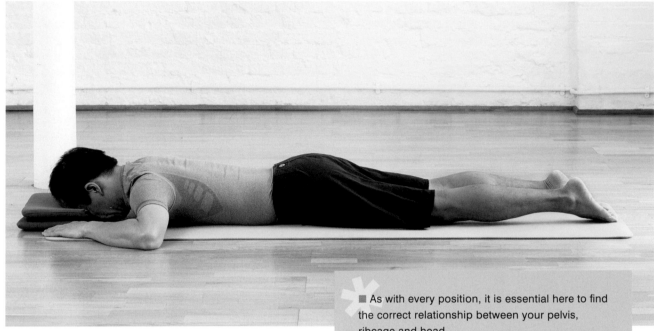

Prone Starting Positions

You will find a variety of prone positions in the book. The arm and leg positions will vary.

✽ Caution: if you have back problems or osteoporosis, you may be more comfortable with a flat folded towel placed under your abdomen. ✽

Lie on your front and position your arms and legs as follows:

■ Create a diamond shape with the arms; place the fingertips together, palms down on the mat and open your elbows. Rest your forehead on your folded hands. If you prefer, rest your forehead on a pillow and place your hands on either side, as shown.

■ Place your legs hip-width apart and parallel. You may place a pillow under your shins if this helps.

✽ ■ As with every position, it is essential here to find the correct relationship between your pelvis, ribcage and head.

■ Allow your hips to open fully and ensure that your weight is evenly distributed across the front of your pelvis. Neither tuck your tailbone under, nor stick it out; in other words, avoid flattening or arching your lower spine.

■ Your lower spine should feel lengthened. If there is any discomfort in your lower spine, then you may place a very small, flat cushion or folded towel under your abdomen to help support your spine.

■ Maintain a connection between the front of your lower ribcage and the top of your pelvis; focus on the heaviness of your ribs releasing into the mat.

■ Allow your chest to be open and although your shoulders should feel released, allow your collar bones to widen.

■ Lengthen your neck while maintaining its natural curve and ensure your focus is directed down, with your chin neither tucked in nor lifted up.

■ Feel your shoulder blades wide in the upper back, and your collarbones open in the front of the chest.

Side-lying Starting Positions

You will find a variety of Side-lying Starting Positions in the book. The head, arm and leg positions vary.

Either: Lie on your side with your knees bent, your feet in line with your spine. Line up hip over hip, knee over knee, shoulder over shoulder. To help check you are straight you can line your torso up with the back edge of your mat.

Or: Bend both knees in front of you so that your hips and knees are bent at a right angle. If you wish, you may place a pillow between your knees to bring your knees, ankles and feet in line with your hips as shown. This is particularly helpful if you have hip or back problems.

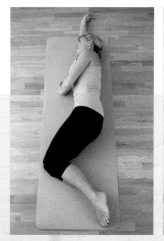 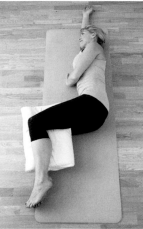

■ Avoid rolling your body forwards or tipping back. Imagine that you are lying in between two planes of glass and stack yourself accordingly.

■ Correctly align your pelvis and spine in neutral, allowing for the natural curves of the spine to be present.

■ Lengthen both sides of your waist equally; this is essential in side-lying as it is very easy to allow the lower side of your spine to dip down towards the mat and for your spine to collapse.

■ Whether your head is supported by your outstretched arm or a cushion, ensure that it is raised sufficiently to align your head and neck with your upper spine. If your head is dropped too low or raised too high, it will affect the position and movement of the rest of your body.

The arm position will vary according to the exercise, but please ensure that you use an appropriate number of cushions/towels to keep your head in alignment with your neck and spine.

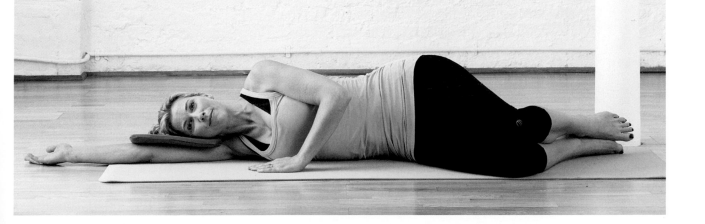

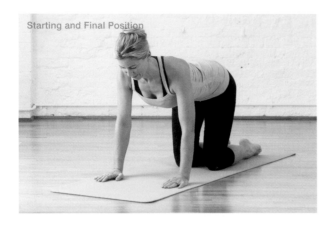

Starting and Final Position

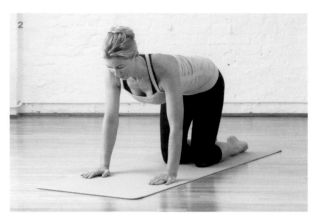

2

Four-Point Kneeling
You cannot just rest in this position, you need to be active!

✱ Caution: take advice with knee problems and avoid if you have recently had breast surgery. Take advice 'going south' if you have osteoporosis or back problems. ✱

Starting Position
Kneel on the mat on all fours. Position your hands directly underneath your shoulders and your knees directly beneath your hips.

■ In this position, it is essential to maintain a good abdominal connection to avoid your pelvis and spine collapsing down towards the mat.

■ The tilting of your pelvis should be small and achieved with ease. The rest of your spine will react slightly, but do not overexaggerate this.

■ Although the movements should be controlled, they should also feel free and released.

■ Fully lengthen your arms, but avoid locking your elbows.

■ Keep your chest and the front of your shoulders open and avoid any tension in your neck area.

Action
The Compass – to find the neutral position of the pelvis and lumbar spine:

1 Breathe in, preparing your body to move. Lengthen your spine.

2 Breathe out as you tilt your pelvis backwards (to north – the pubic bone moves forwards), allowing your lower back to round slightly (flex).

3 Breathe in and lengthen the spine and tilt the pelvis forwards (to south – the pubic bone moves backwards), allowing your lower back to arch slightly (extend).

Repeat 3 times, then find the mid-position in between these two extremes, where your pelvis is neutral. This position is lengthened and level, neither tucked nor arched. Allow for the natural curvature of the lumbar spine.

To help encourage awareness of the correct position of the shoulder blades on the ribcage try the following:

4 Breathe in and, keeping your elbows straight, gently draw your shoulder blades together (retracting them). Your upper spine will lower slightly towards the mat.

5 Breathe out as you allow your shoulder blades to glide apart on your ribcage (at the back). Your upper spine will round slightly.

Repeat 3 times, then find the mid-position of the shoulder blades in between these two extremes. Allow for the natural curvature of the upper spine and neck. Lengthen the whole spine from the crown of your head to your tailbone.

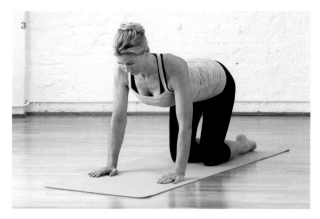

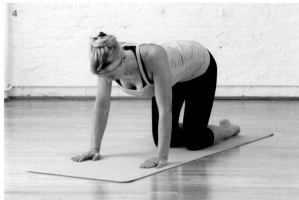

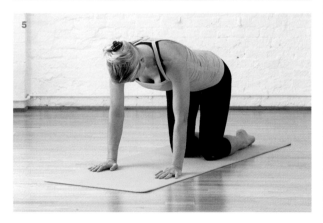

High Kneeling

✳ Caution: avoid this if you have knee problems or simply find this position uncomfortable. ✳

High kneel on your mat. You will need a lightly padded mat to protect your knees.

Have your knees hip-width apart. You may place a small cushion between the thighs. (The cushion should be about hip-width in thickness.)

Your lower legs should be parallel and hip-width apart. Ensure that your weight falls not just through the knees, but through the length of both shin bones evenly.

■ Lengthen up through the spine.

■ Also lengthen your waist equally on both sides.

■ Allow your ribcage to relax and be positioned directly above the pelvis, neither swaying backwards nor slumping forwards.

■ Feel your shoulder blades wide in the upper back, and your collarbones open in the front of the chest. Soften your breastbone.

■ Allow your arms to hang freely in the shoulder sockets. Feel space underneath the armpits and a sense of length and weight through the hands.

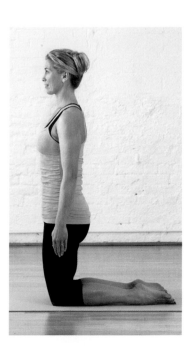

■ Release your neck and allow your head to balance freely on top of the spine; sense the crown of the head lengthening up to the ceiling.

■ Relax your jaw muscles and focus directly forwards.

Standing Alignment

We are aiming for 80 per cent of your body weight to be balanced over the arches of your feet. This is ideal as it reduces the load on the joints created by being upright against gravity and also enables you to cope with walking on different types of surfaces.

We have no fewer than 17 watchpoints to help you to stand well! This is because standing tall is a dynamic exercise rather than a 'position', and it requires you to be active. As your core muscles become more efficient through your Pilates practice, you will find standing and sitting tall effortless and you will be able to find and maintain good posture easily.

Starting Position

Stand tall on the floor (not on your mat) and place your feet hip-width apart in a natural stance, neither turned out nor in a rigid parallel position. Allow your arms to lengthen down by your sides. Have a sturdy chair alongside for stability if needed.

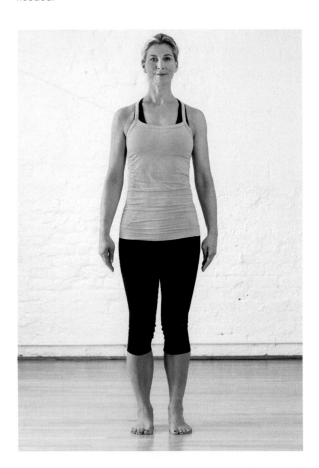

■ Lean forwards slightly from the ankle joints, so that your weight shifts on to the balls of your feet; the heels stay down.

■ Lean backwards slightly from the ankle joints, so that your weight shifts on to the heels; the toes should be lengthened and without tension.

■ Place your weight in the centre of the feet, over the arches, and notice that there is a triangle of connection with the floor: the base of the big toe, the little toe and the centre of the heel. The toes should be active.

■ Lengthen your legs. Allow your knees to soften.

■ Tilt your pelvis forwards slightly (so that your lower back arches slightly).

■ Pass through neutral, then slightly tilt your pelvis backwards, slightly rounding your lower back.

■ Return your pelvis to a neutral, mid position.

■ Lengthen your waist equally on both sides.

■ Find your centre by gently recruiting your pelvic floor and the deep abdominal muscles.

■ Allow your ribcage to relax and be positioned directly above the pelvis, neither swaying backwards, nor slumping forwards.

■ Feel your shoulder blades wide in the upper back, and your collarbones open in the front of the chest. Soften your breastbone.

■ Allow your arms to hang freely in the shoulder sockets. Feel space underneath the armpits and a sense of length and weight through the hands.

■ Release your neck and allow your head to balance freely on top of the spine, sense the crown of the head lengthening up to the ceiling.

■ Relax your jaw muscles and focus forwards.

■ Maintain a sense of what is happening in your lower body and be aware of your feet on the floor.

■ Breathe naturally into the ribcage.

■ This position should not feel forced or held. You should feel you are growing upwards dynamically.

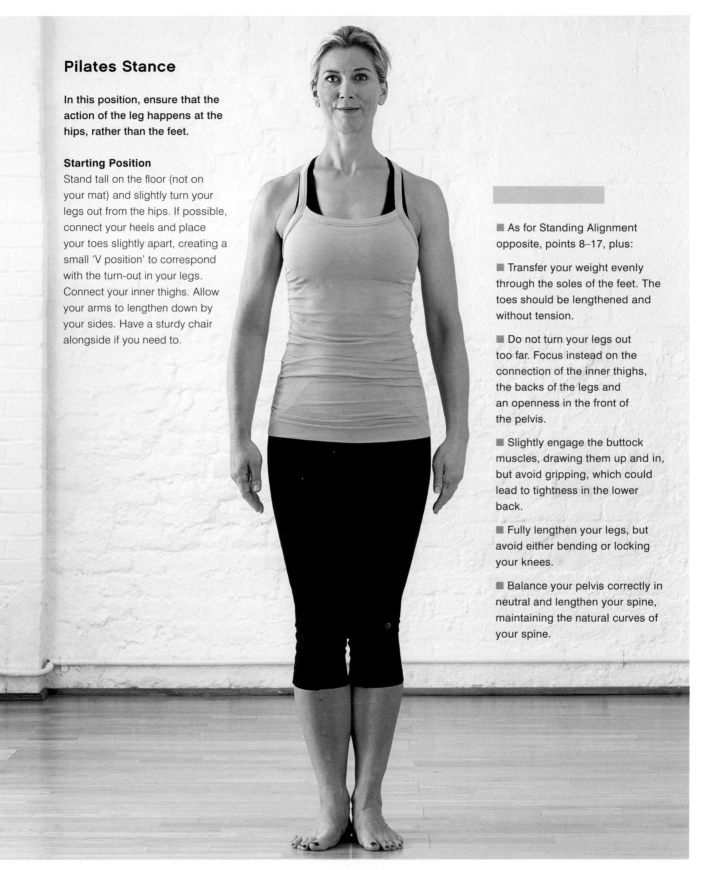

Pilates Stance

In this position, ensure that the action of the leg happens at the hips, rather than the feet.

Starting Position
Stand tall on the floor (not on your mat) and slightly turn your legs out from the hips. If possible, connect your heels and place your toes slightly apart, creating a small 'V position' to correspond with the turn-out in your legs. Connect your inner thighs. Allow your arms to lengthen down by your sides. Have a sturdy chair alongside if you need to.

■ As for Standing Alignment opposite, points 8–17, plus:

■ Transfer your weight evenly through the soles of the feet. The toes should be lengthened and without tension.

■ Do not turn your legs out too far. Focus instead on the connection of the inner thighs, the backs of the legs and an openness in the front of the pelvis.

■ Slightly engage the buttock muscles, drawing them up and in, but avoid gripping, which could lead to tightness in the lower back.

■ Fully lengthen your legs, but avoid either bending or locking your knees.

■ Balance your pelvis correctly in neutral and lengthen your spine, maintaining the natural curves of your spine.

BREATHING

Breathing is an automatic process that we rarely think about. Most of us breathe far too shallowly and much faster than we need to. If you use mainly the upper part of your chest to breathe you are only using a fraction of your capacity for air. If you breathe more rapidly, you take in a new breath before emptying your lungs of the stale air. This stale air is then mixed with the fresh air, decreasing your supply of oxygen and thus your energy.

We will be using different types of breathing in the programme with different end goals in mind. We will use lateral thoracic breathing (Scarf Breathing, see below) for most of the exercises, but also deep abdominal breathing later in the programme to encourage release of the pelvic floor (p. 177). When building your Pilates skills you will need to breathe well in order to learn how to stabilise.

Remember too that you must think about good alignment before you try a breathing exercise, as efficient breathing relies on good posture. It is very difficult to breathe well with a hunched posture, since your ribs are compressed and your thoracic cavity and main breathing muscle – your diaphragm – are restricted.

We want to focus on a deeper, more rhythmic way of breathing where the diaphragm is encouraged to move up and down more which, in turn, allows the thoracic cavity (the area within the ribcage) to expand fully. A full inhalation followed by a deep exhalation helps increase your capacity to inhale new fresh air.

Although you won't be able to feel the diaphragm, it may help to visualise this big dome-shaped muscle separating the thoracic cavity horizontally from the abdominal cavity. You will also need to locate your lungs, which are situated towards the back of the ribcage. To help focus on this area, try the following exercise:

'Therefore, above all, learn how to breathe correctly.'

Return to Life Through Contrology, **Joseph Pilates**

Scarf Breathing
(lateral thoracic breathing)
The scarf gives you sensory feedback to help you feel your ribcage expanding and closing with your breath.

1 Sit or stand tall and wrap a scarf or stretch band around the lower part of your ribs, crossing it over at the front. Hold the opposite ends of the scarf and gently pull it tight.

The Inhalation
2 As you breathe in, focus on the back and the sides of the ribcage where your lungs are located. Like balloons swelling gradually with air, your lungs will expand and widen the walls of your ribcage. Do not be tempted to force this inhalation, as you will only create tension. You should feel the scarf tightening as your ribs expand.

It is not only the lungs filling up that expands your ribcage, but also the descent of the diaphragm as it lowers into your abdominal area which will, in turn, extend outwards.

Breathe in through your nose and keep your shoulders relaxed.

The Exhalation

As you breathe out, feel the air gently being pushed out fully, as if from the very bottom of your lungs, eventually exiting your body via your mouth with a deep sigh.

Your diaphragm will begin to rise and you should feel your ribcage reactively beginning to close as your lungs empty. It should also feel easier to connect to your core muscles, which will be our next task (pp. 38–39).

Do not puff your cheeks or purse your lips, as this will tense the neck, jaw and face, and waste energy.

The Timing

The timing of the breath is also important to your Pilates practice. We use certain breathing patterns to help facilitate better movement. However, you may find this timing difficult at first, especially if you are used to other fitness regimes. When you first start to practise the exercises, you may focus on controlling the movements, then, when you have those under control, you can add in controlling your breathing. Most importantly, do not hold your breath or force it in any way.

Make sure that you do not over-breathe. Your breathing should be at a natural, easy pace. If you need to take an extra breath or change the timing of the breath, please do so.

Remember:

■ Never hold your breath when exercising.
■ Breathe fully, but naturally, and without force.
■ Breath initiates each movement and will help you to improve the flow and the enjoyable ease of your movement.
■ Certain breath patterns will help particular movements, so if a movement is feeling forced or uncomfortable, check firstly that you are breathing and secondly that you are breathing correctly to help facilitate the movement.

There are many more breathing exercises for you to try later in the book (see Respiratory Health pp. 166–71 and Women's and Men's Health pp. 175–77).

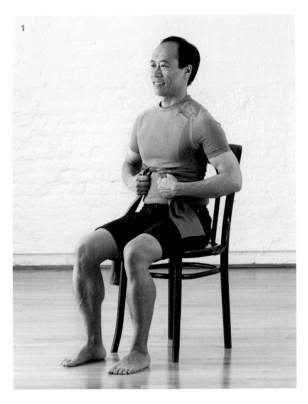

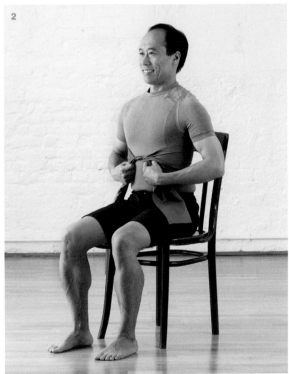

CENTRING

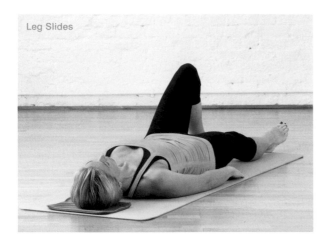

Leg Slides

Centring is another of the key principles that firmly underpins the Pilates method. The term 'centring' encompasses many of the popular and widely talked about concepts associated with 'stability training'. So what do we mean here by 'stability'?

In general terms we would call an object stable if it can cope with the demands placed on it. A stable chair is one that is built to carry the weight of the person sitting on it and can also remain upright if it is, for example, knocked. But stability can also be applied to moving objects, such as a bicycle.

In Pilates, stability might best be viewed as the ability to maintain control of the movements you perform, stopping undesired movements while allowing the desired movements to be performed with maximum efficiency. This means that we cannot consider stability without considering mobility. Stability is not just about holding a joint still; the joints involved in any movement also need to be controlled.

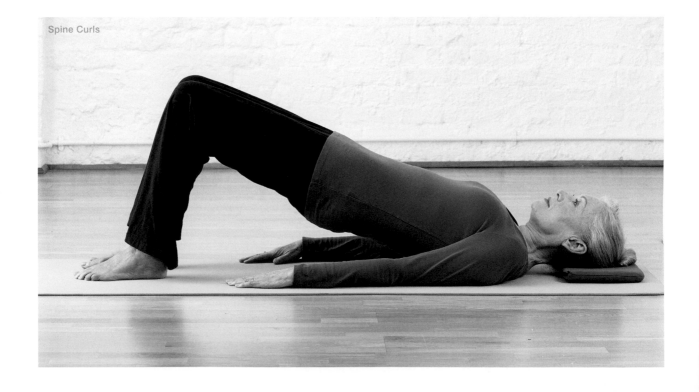

Spine Curls

Leg Slides (p. 42) are a perfect example. They require the pelvis and spine to remain still while the legs move, so the stability of the spine and pelvis is challenged while the leg is moving. In contrast, for Spine Curls (p. 58), the pelvis and spine should move while the legs are still; you are controlling the rolling of the spine, bone by bone. This demands a level of pelvic and spinal stability to prevent any undesired movements such as twisting or hiking up on one side.

With a clearer understanding of what we mean by stability, we can now look at 'core stability', which relates to what Joseph Pilates called centring. Core stability is being able to stabilise and control the position of the different segments of the body; that is, the pelvis, spine, ribcage, shoulders and head. Gaining stability in this core area provides a strong and stable base of support from which all Pilates movements are initiated. To do this we have to train the core muscles, and these will vary depending on the movement you are doing. As a beginner in Pilates you will usually learn how to activate the core muscles while your trunk is in a still position. This is simply because it is easier for you to feel what you are doing and control it. But you will not be staying still for long.

We have already noted that there are many different schools of Pilates, each with its own preferred way of describing how to engage your core muscles. The words that are used are not really important – rather, it is the feeling of the 'connection to inner control' that they try to convey. This connection needs to be found and used as needed to control your movements. And although much of the stability process is dealt with on a subconscious level, it is also possible to train and improve stability throughout the body with conscious control. This is what we'll be doing here.

Through Pilates, we hope to prepare your body, so that it will subconsciously react to any demand placed on it by automatically using the deep core muscles. Pilates is based on the principle that by practising control over movements during a Pilates session, and repeating good movements, you pattern or ingrain these movements into your mind and body, thus improving the quality of your movements as you go about your daily activities.

The Dimmer Switch
When you are doing Pilates exercises, we encourage you to gently engage your deep stabilising muscles and keep them engaged at an appropriate level to control your movements. But what is an 'appropriate level'?

One of the most common mistakes made when doing 'stability training' style exercises is over-recruitment of the core muscles. The trick is only to engage your deep core as much as you need to control the movement. No more, no less. We call this the Dimmer Switch approach – you are constantly adjusting the level to match the demands that are placed on the body.

If you do not have back problems or osteoporosis, you can try comparing the Single- and Double-knee Fold exercises (pp. 44–45) as they clearly show the relationship between the amount of centring required and the physical demands of the exercise being performed. When you try them, notice how you only need to engage your deep muscles gently for the Single-knee Fold, whereas you have to 'turn up the dimmer switch' and engage your core more strongly as you attempt to lift the second leg in the Double-knee version.

Once you have mastered connecting to your centre with the exercises on pp40–53, you can apply what you have learned to all the other exercises in this book.

It may be that as you become proficient at doing the exercises you will not need to actively engage your core; as you learn to control your alignment through movement, they will automatically engage.

Finding your centre – the Wind Zip and Abdominal Hollowing

The focus of this exercise is simply to learn how to feel and connect to your centre.

Starting Position

Sit upright on a chair. Place your feet on the floor, hip-width apart. Make sure that your weight is even on both sitting bones and that your spine is lengthened in neutral.

Action

1 Breathe in to prepare, and lengthen through your spine.

2 Breathe out as you gently squeeze your back passage (anus), as if trying to prevent yourself from passing wind, then bring this feeling forwards towards your pubic bone, as if trying to stop yourself from passing water. Continue to gently draw these pelvic-floor muscles up inside. You should feel your abdominals automatically begin to hollow. Imagine you are engaging an internal zip from back to front and up inside.

3 Maintain this core connection and breathe normally for 5 breaths; you should feel that your ribs are still free to move. Then relax.

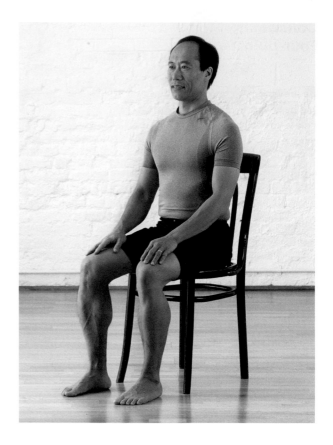

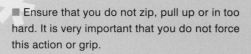

■ Ensure that you do not zip, pull up or in too hard. It is very important that you do not force this action or grip.

■ Make sure that you keep your buttock muscles relaxed.

■ Keep your chest and the front of your shoulders open and avoid any tension in your neck area.

■ Keep your breathing smooth and evenly paced; ensuring that your ribcage and abdominal area are still able to expand with your in-breath is a good sign that you haven't overengaged.

■ If you lose any of the connections, relax and start again from the beginning.

To remind you to connect your centre through this zip-and-abdominal hollowing action during the exercises, you will see the following phrase: 'Use an appropriate level of core connection to control your alignment and movements.'

Please remember the 'Dimmer Switch' (p. 39) and be aware of when you may need to engage these muscles more or less. The goal is to stay in control of your movements. If you find 'the zip' part difficult, please do not worry – it will come eventually.

Try the pelvic-floor exercises on pp. 175-177 to help your awareness of these important muscles.

If you still find the zip too difficult, focus on simply scooping the abdominals, drawing them lightly back towards the spine. At the end of the day, what matters is that you are in control of your body as you move to avoid injury. This will become automatic as you practise more.

Connecting to your core muscles: Four-point Kneeling

We are all individuals and sometimes what works for one person may not work for another person. Trying to isolate your core muscles in a variety of positions and ways is a good way to find out what works for you.

✳ Caution: take advice if you have a knee problem or have recently had a breast operation. ✳

Starting Position

Kneel on all fours on the mat. Position your hands directly underneath your shoulders and your knees directly beneath your hips. Gently rock your pelvis and settle in the mid-position where your pelvis is neutral. This position is lengthened and level, neither tucked nor arched. Allow for the natural curvature of the lumbar spine. Find the mid-position of the shoulder blades, allowing for the natural curvature of the upper spine and neck. Lengthen the whole spine from the crown of the head to your tailbone.

Action

1 Breathe in to prepare.

2 Breathe out as you gently squeeze your back passage (anus), as if trying to prevent yourself from passing wind, then bringing this feeling forwards towards your pubic bone. Now draw these muscles up inside until you feel your abdominals automatically begin to hollow.

3 Maintain this connection and breathe normally for 5 breaths. Then release, ensuring that your abdominals and ribs are still able to move with your breath.

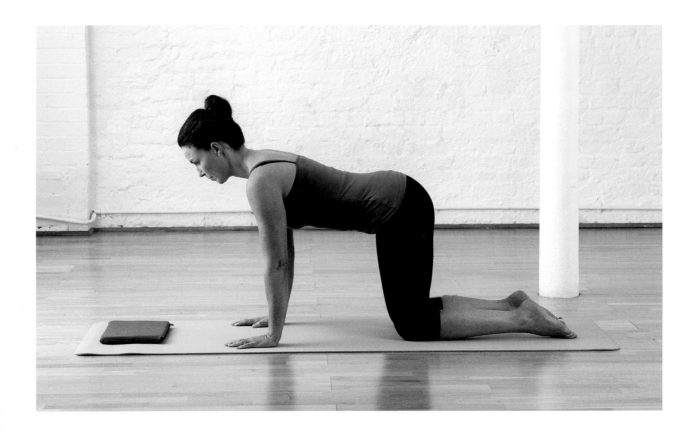

Challenging your core: Leg Slides, Knee Openings, Knee Folds

Hopefully, by now you feel confident in how to place your body in good alignment, how to breathe laterally and how to connect to your centre. Now it is time to challenge your ability to control these fundamentals. In the following exercises, you will learn how to move your limbs while keeping the pelvis and spine still. Later on we will challenge your core in other ways.

This group of exercises helps you focus on maintaining a stable relationship between the pelvis and spine, while promoting independent movement of your leg at your hip joint. You can vary which exercises you practise each session, but the Starting Position is the same for all four.

Starting Position

The Relaxation Position, arms lengthened alongside you on the mat. Or, initially, you may want to place your hands on your pelvis to check for unwanted movement.

Use an appropriate level of core connection to control your alignment and movements.

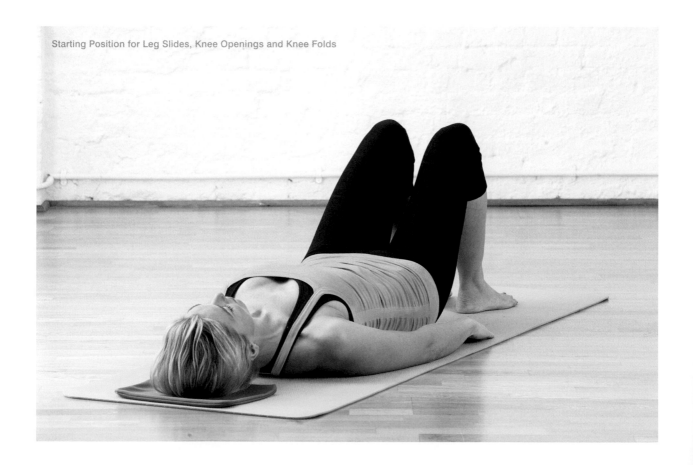

Starting Position for Leg Slides, Knee Openings and Knee Folds

Action for Leg Slides

1 Breathe in, widening your ribcage to prepare to move.

2 Breathe out, as you slide one leg away along the floor in line with your hip, keeping your pelvis and spine stable and in neutral.

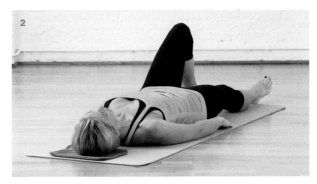

3 Breathe in as you draw your leg back in line with your hip to the Starting Position.

Repeat 5 times with each leg.

Action for Knee Openings

Use an appropriate level of core connection to control your alignment and movements.

1 Breathe in to prepare to move.

2 Breathe out as you allow one knee to open slowly to the side; keep the foot down on the mat, but allow it to roll to the outer edge. Open as far as you can without disturbing the pelvis.

3 Breathe in as you bring the knee back to the Starting Position.

Repeat 5 times with each leg.

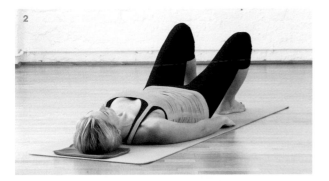

On all exercises...

■ Keep your pelvis and spine still and centred throughout. Focus on your leg moving in isolation from the rest of your body.

■ Focus on your waist remaining long and even on both sides as you slide your leg in and out.

■ Remain still in the supporting leg, without tension.

■ Keep your foot in contact with the floor and in line with your hip.

■ Keep your chest and the front of your shoulders open and release any tension in your neck area.

■ Alternate which leg you start with each time you workout.

For Knee Openings...

As before plus:

■ Focus especially on not allowing your pelvis to rock to either side.

■ Keep your supporting leg correctly aligned and still; do not allow it to open away from the working leg.

Action for Single-knee Folds

Use an appropriate level of core connection to control your alignment and movements.

1 Breathe in to prepare your body to move.

2 Breathe out as you lift your right foot off the mat and fold the knee up towards your body. Allow the weight of the leg to drop down into your hip socket and remain grounded in your pelvis and long in your spine.

3 Breathe in, maintain the position and stay centred.

4 Breathe out as you slowly return the leg back down and your foot to the mat.

Repeat 5 times with each leg.

For Single-knee Folds...

As on p.43 plus:

■ Keep your pelvis and spine still and centred throughout. Focus on your leg moving in isolation from the rest of your body. Be especially careful as you begin to lift your leg.

■ Fold your knee in as far as you can without disturbing the pelvis and losing neutral.

■ Fold your knee directly in line with your hip joint.

■ Avoid cheating by pressing down with your other foot.

For Double-knee Folds...

■ As above, but ensure that you use an appropriate amount of core connection, bearing in mind that lifting and lowering your second knee will require much more stability.

■ Continue to breathe; do not forget!

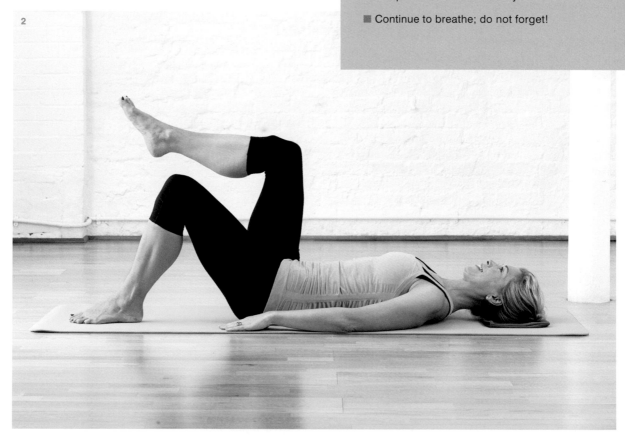

2

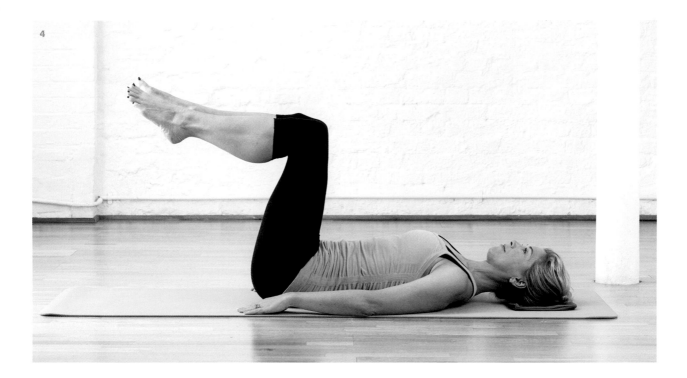

4

Action for Double-knee Folds
Note: this is an advanced exercise. We have included it here because it is a fundamental pelvic-stability exercise. However, it is by no means easy to perform well and should not be attempted until you are confident with all the previous exercises in this section.

Use an appropriate level of core connection to control your alignment and movements.

✳ Caution: avoid this version if you have osteoporosis or back problems, but take advice as to whether you may do the variation. ✳

1 Breathe in, preparing your body to move.

2 Breathe out as you fold one knee in. Remain grounded in your pelvis and long in your spine.

3 Breathe in, maintain the position and stay centred.

4 Breathe out as you increase your connection to your centre and fold your left knee up and towards you.

5 Breathe in, maintaining your position and staying centred

as your pelvis remains grounded in neutral.

6 Breathe out as you slowly lower your right foot to the mat. Do not allow the abdominals to bulge or your pelvis to lose neutral.

7 Breathe out as you slowly return the left leg back down and your foot to the mat.

Repeat 6 times, alternating sides.

Moving on... When you are happy that you can do this exercise easily with control, you may raise and lower each leg, still one at a time, but on a single out-breath.

Variation: Double-knee Folds place quite a strain on the lumbar spine, which is why it may be contraindicated for some conditions such as osteoporosis. You may, however, be able to try this version as your hands will help support the weight of the legs, thus reducing the load.

Follow all the directions above, but as one knee folds in, place one hand on the leg, supporting it lightly under the thigh, and then do the same for the second knee. Take care not to round your upper back.

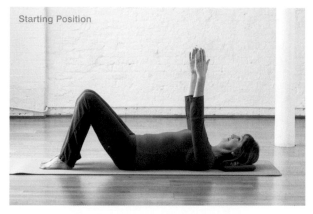
Starting Position

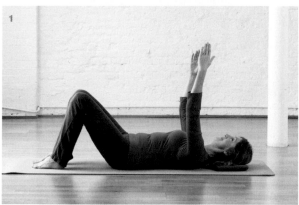
1

■ Keep your pelvis and spine stable and still throughout.

■ Keep your neck long and free from tension and your head still and heavy throughout.

■ Use the breathing pattern to guide your movements; the inhalation encourages the ribcage to widen and the shoulder blades to glide, the exhalation encourages a release of tension.

■ Fully lengthen your arms, but avoid locking your elbows.

Shoulder Drops

So far we have been challenging your core control with the lower limbs. Now it's time to try the upper limbs. But first we need to get your shoulders organised and in the best place. Shoulder Drops are great for this, as well as for helping release tension from around the shoulders and neck by mobilising the shoulder blades. They also develop your awareness of the arms' connection to the back of the ribcage via the shoulder girdle.

Starting Position

The Relaxation Position. Raise both arms vertically above your chest, shoulder-width apart, with your palms facing one another.

Use an appropriate level of core connection to control your alignment and movements.

Action

1 Breathe in as you reach one arm up towards the ceiling, peeling the shoulder blade away from the mat.

2 Breathe out as you gently release the arm back down, returning the shoulder blade back to the mat.

Repeat up to 10 times, alternating arms.

Variation

Reach and release both arms at the same time.

Ribcage Closure

This exercise challenges your core stability from the top end. Your primary goal is to stay in control of the position of your ribcage and upper spine. The exercise also improves shoulder mobility.

Starting Position

The Relaxation Position – arms lengthened down by your sides, palms facing inwards. Take a moment to notice the weight of your ribs, pelvis and head on the mat. This shouldn't change during the exercise.

Use an appropriate level of core connection to control your alignment and movements.

Action

1 Breathe in and raise both arms to shoulder height, palms facing each other.

2 Breathe out as you reach both arms overhead towards the floor. Keep your neck long and encourage the softening and the closing of the ribcage (keep your ribs connected and don't allow them to pop up). Keep your spine still and stable.

3 Breathe in as you return the arms to above your chest. Feel your ribcage heavy and your collarbones open.

4 Breathe out and lower the arms, lengthening as you return them to your sides. Repeat up to 10 times.

■ Note that unless you are very flexible, it is unlikely that your arms will reach the floor behind you. Ear level is normal. If your range of movement does allow your arms to reach all the way to the floor, don't allow them to relax there.

■ Be particularly careful not to allow your upper spine to arch as you reach your arms overhead.

■ Try not to hunch your shoulders; allow them to move naturally and without tension.

■ Lengthen your arms; avoid locking your elbows.

■ Keep your neck long and free from tension.

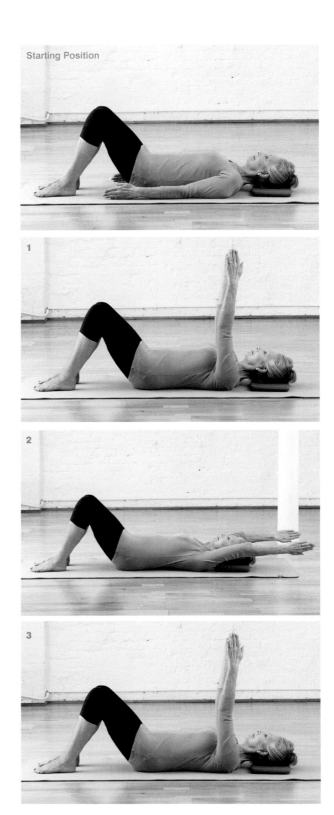

Starting Position

1

2

3

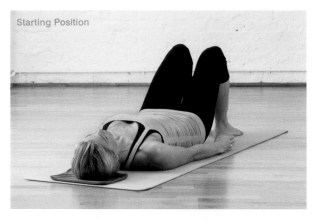

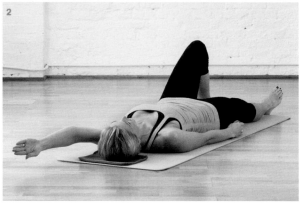

- As you draw the leg back, focus on the back of your thigh rather than the front.

- The ribs stay integrated with your waist as the arm reaches away.

- Think wide and open across your collarbones.

- Maintain the distance between your ears and your shoulders.

- The pelvis stays still and neutral when your leg slides out and when it slides back.

- Slide the leg in a line with the hip. Think of using the back of the thigh rather than the front to bring the leg back.

Starfish

This exercise calls for free, flowing movement away from a strong centre. As your arm moves back, think of what you learned in Ribcage Closure (p. 47). As the leg slides away, think of what you learned in Leg Slides (p. 43)

Starting Position

The Relaxation Position with your arms down by your sides, palms facing your body.

Use an appropriate level of core connection to control your alignment and movements.

Action

1 Breathe in to prepare.

2 Breathe out as you raise one arm back as if to touch the floor behind you. Move the arm as far as you can without disturbing the ribcage or spine. Simultaneously, slide the opposite leg away along the floor in a line with your hip, keeping the pelvis stable.

3 Breathe in and enjoy lengthening away from your strong centre.

4 Breathe out and return the limbs to the Starting Position.

Repeat up to 10 times, alternating arms and legs.

Star Preparation

In this exercise you are in a prone position and you learn how to extend your hip (lift your leg) while keeping a stable pelvis. You will find the Full Star on p. 109 and another version on p. 118.

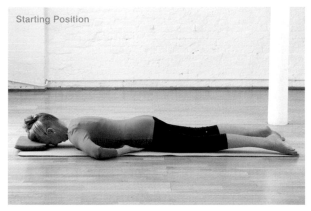
Starting Position

Starting Position

Lie prone. Rest your forehead on a folded towel. Place your fingertips just under your pelvic bones. Your legs are straight, slightly wider than hip-width and turned out from the hips. Or you may have the legs in parallel. Note the pressure on your fingertips. The goal is not to increase or decrease this pressure as the leg lifts. It is not as easy as it sounds.

Use an appropriate level of core connection to control your alignment and movements.

Action

1 Breathe in, preparing your body to move.

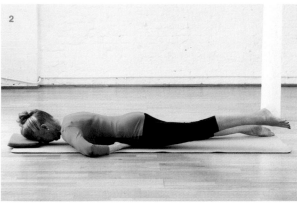
2

2 Breathe out and, maintaining the position and stability of the spine and pelvis, lengthen and lift one leg off the mat. You should not feel any change in the pressure on your fingertips.

3 Breathe in as you lengthen and lower your leg back down to the mat.

Repeat up to 10 times, lifting alternate legs.

■ Keep your core connected to support your lower back.

■ Raise your leg only as high as you can without disturbing the pelvis and spine.

■ Fully lengthen your legs, but avoid locking your knees.

And for the Variation...

■ Lengthen the knee away from the hip joint as you lift.

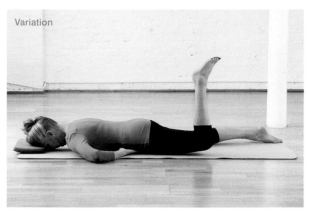
Variation

Variation: Prone Knee Lifts

In this version of the Star, the working knee is bent. This variation is an important exercise for your gluteals, which tend to weaken with age, as it isolates and strengthens them.

Action

Follow all the directions above but with a bent knee. Your hands can be folded under your forehead if you prefer.

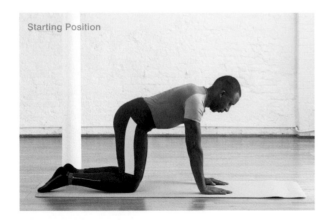

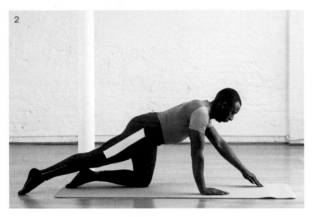

- ■ In this Four-point Kneeling Position, it is essential to maintain a good abdominal connection to prevent your pelvis and spine dipping down towards the mat.

- ■ Focus on the stability and stillness of your pelvis and ribcage, as your leg moves freely and independently in the hip socket.

- ■ Maintain a firm connection of the shoulder blades to the back of your ribcage.

- ■ Keep lengthening both sides of the waist throughout. Try to avoid 'hitching' your pelvis up towards your ribcage.

- ■ Maintain correct alignment of your head and neck with your upper spine and keep your neck free from tension.

Table-top Preparation

This exercise primarily challenges the stability of the entire spine and shoulder girdle in a Four-point Kneeling Position (p. 32) while trying to find independent, free and flowing movement of the legs. This version is the ideal preparation for the more challenging Full Table-top (p. 111) where you lift your opposite arm and leg.

✳ Caution: avoid this exercise if you have knee problems or have recently had a breast operation. ✳

Starting Position

Adopt the Four-point Kneeling Position.

Use an appropriate level of core connection to control your alignment and movements.

Action

1 Breathe in, preparing your body to move, and lengthen your spine.

2 Breathe out, maintaining a still and stable pelvis and spine, slide one leg behind you, directly in line with your hip. Your softly pointed foot will remain in contact with the mat. At the same time, lengthen the opposite arm away from the shoulder, keeping the hand in contact with the mat.

3 Breathe in as you maintain the position.

4 Breathe out as you bend the knee and slide the arm and leg back to the Starting Position.

Repeat up to 8 times, alternating opposite arm and leg.

Side-lying Stability: Oyster

Arguably one of the most important exercises in this book, Oyster helps strengthen your deep gluteals which help stabilise your pelvis. If that doesn't motivate you, just think of it as firming up your buttocks! You may need a flat cushion or folded towel.

✳ Caution: if you have had a recent hip replacement, move gently within your pain-free zone and with control. ✳

Starting Position

Side-lying on your left side, in a straight line, stack your shoulders, hips and ankles. Pelvis and spine should remain in neutral. Lengthen your left arm underneath your head and in line with your spine, palm up; you will probably need a flat cushion or folded towel to keep your head in line with your spine. Place your left hand on the mat in front of your ribcage and bend your elbow to help lightly support your position. Bend both knees and draw your feet back, so that your heels are aligned with the back of your pelvis. Place a cushion between your knees.

Use an appropriate level of core connection to control your alignment and movements.

Action

1 Breathe in, preparing your body to move.

2 Breathe out as you open your top knee, keeping your feet connected. This 'turn-out' movement will come from your hip joint. Keep your pelvis still and stable.

3 Breathe in and, with control, return your leg to the Starting Position.

Repeat up to 10 times and then repeat on the other side.

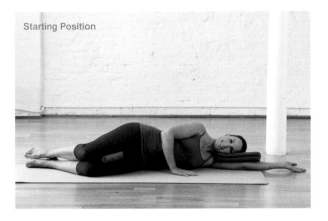

Starting Position

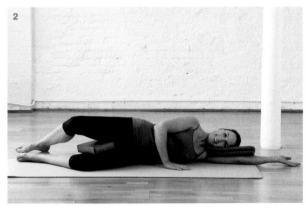

■ Ensure correct alignment in your side-lying starting position: shoulder above shoulder, hip above hip and knee above knee.

■ To help reach the right muscles, try gently squeezing your heels together. Make sure that both heels squeeze evenly.

■ Open your top leg only as far as you can without disturbing the position of your pelvis.

■ Keep lengthening both sides of the waist throughout.

■ The top arm is positioned to help support you, but avoid placing too much weight on it.

■ Keep your chest open, and your focus directly ahead of you.

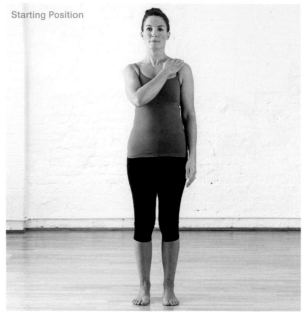

Starting Position

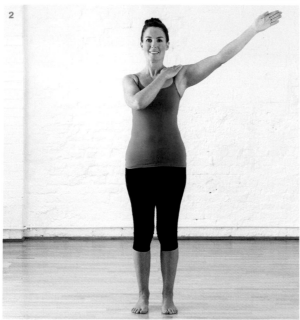

2

■ Keep a sense of openness in the upper body.

■ Do not allow your upper body to shift to the side; keep centred. Do not over-elevate your shoulders.

■ Keep your arms lengthened but not bent; ensure that the movement comes only from the shoulders.

Floating Arms

So far the exercises we have practised have started in the Relaxation Position. But our programme needs to reflect daily life, much of which is spent upright. The change in position will mean that gravity has a different impact on your body: when you are standing, achieving control of the relationship between your main body weights – your head, ribcage and pelvis – is more challenging.

Many of us have a tendency to overuse the upper part of our shoulders – it's why these muscles can get really tense. This simple exercise will help you find a way of lifting your arm that doesn't overuse these muscles.

As you raise your arm, think of this order of movement: first, just your arm moves up and out, then you will feel the shoulder blade start to move, coiling down and around the back of the ribcage. Finally, the collarbone (clavicle) will lift.

Starting Position

Sit or stand tall, remembering the instructions on p.34. Place your right hand on your left shoulder. Feel your collarbone – you are going to try to keep it still for the first part of the movement, your hand checking that the upper part of your shoulder remains 'quiet' for as long as possible. Very often this part will overwork, so think of it staying soft and released.

Use an appropriate level of core connection to control your alignment and movements.

Action

1 Breathe in to prepare, and lengthen up through the spine.

2 Breathe out as you slowly begin to raise the arm, reaching wide out of the shoulder blades like a bird's wing. Imagine the middle finger of your hand leading the arm – the arm following the hand as it floats upwards. Keep your arm just in front of your shoulders so that it remains within your peripheral vision; allow it to rotate naturally within the shoulder socket as it lifts.

3 Breathe in as you lower the arm to your side, following the same pathway.

Repeat 3 times with each arm.

Standing Stability:
Standing On One Leg

Think of this as a standing Knee-fold (p. 44). This exercise is important for balance as well as stability. It can easily be incorporated into your everyday activities – try cleaning your teeth standing on one leg (say 90 seconds for each leg, or stand on one leg as you brush the upper teeth, then the other for the lower).

✻ Caution: take advice if you have balance, vestibular or knee, ankle or foot problems. ✻

Starting Position
Stand tall on the floor (not on your mat), feet hip-width apart. Have a sturdy chair alongside you.

Use an appropriate level of core connection to control your alignment and movements.

Action
1 Breathe in, preparing your body to move, and lengthen your spine.

2 Breathe out; transfer your weight on to your right leg and, keeping the pelvis as level as possible, bend your left knee to lift your foot slightly off the floor and draw your leg up and in towards your torso.

3 Breathe in as you hold this lengthened and stable position, feeling the crown of your head reaching away from your grounded right foot.

4 Breathe out, return your left leg back to the standing position and evenly distribute your weight through both feet.

Repeat up to 5 times on each side, alternating legs.

Variation
For a greater challenge, start with your feet together.

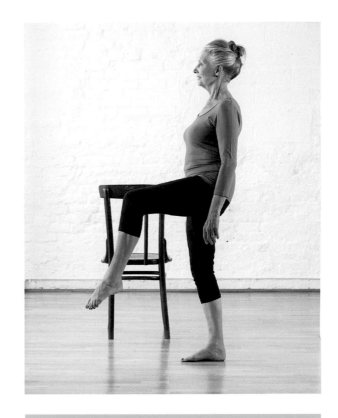

✻
■ Maintain neutral pelvis and spine throughout. Keep lengthening both sides of the waist and try to avoid 'hitching' up one side of your pelvis towards your ribcage.

■ Keep your weight balanced evenly through the entire surface area of your foot. Do not allow your foot to roll in or out or scrunch your toes up.

■ Fully lengthen your supporting leg, but avoid locking the knee.

■ Maintain the parallel alignment of your supporting leg; ensure that your knee remains facing forwards.

■ Release your neck and allow the head to balance freely on top of the spine; sense the crown of the head lengthening up to the ceiling.

MOBILITY

We need to be stable both when we are still and when we are in motion – stability does not equal stillness. The exercises we have introduced so far focused on maintaining a still, stable relationship between ribcage, pelvis and spine while your limbs moved. Now it's time to challenge your ability to control this relationship with movement.

Joseph Pilates wrote that he wanted the spine to move in a 'synchronous and smooth manner'. The spine should be both stable and mobile, able to articulate freely, vertebra by vertebra, in what is often referred to as segmental control. Although there is very little movement between adjacent vertebrae, it is vital to maintain this subtle motion, the cumulative effect along the length of the spine being almost snakelike.

In order to go about our daily activities, we need to be able to bend forwards (flexion of the spine), backwards (extension of the spine), to the side (lateral flexion of the spine) and to twist (rotation of the spine), and most of our activities are combinations of these movements. Pilates exercises will help you learn how to control and articulate your spine segment by segment, bone by bone, through these various movements. If you plan your own workouts, always include all these movements to keep your sessions balanced.

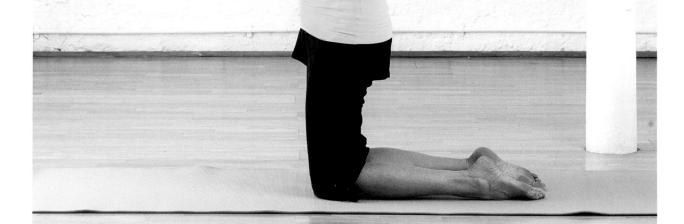

Rotation

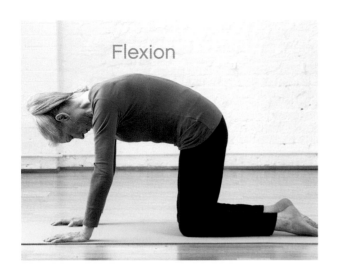

Flexion

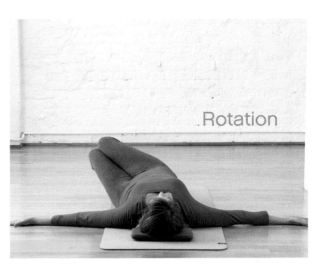

Rotation

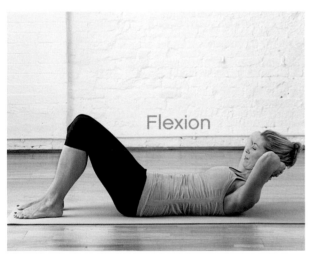

Flexion

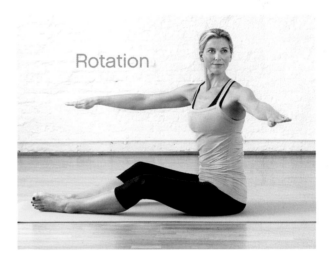

Rotation

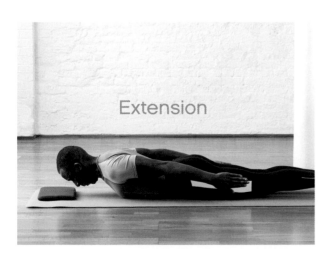

Extension

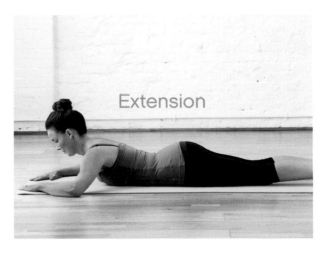

Extension

SPINAL FLEXION

Seated C-curve

This is not always an easy exercise to get right, but it is a very valuable one. It teaches you how to lengthen your spine in a forward C-curve. This skill is used again and again in Pilates, for example in the Cat (opposite).

✳ Caution: take care to elongate your spine in the C-curve if you have been diagnosed with osteoporosis. No collapsing! ✳

Starting Position

Sit tall on the mat. Have your knees bent, feet hip-width apart, the soles of your feet planted firmly on the mat. Place your hands behind your thighs, your elbows open and wide. If you find it difficult to sit with a neutral pelvis and spine in this position, sit on a cushion or rolled-up towel to attain the correct alignment.

Use an appropriate level of core connection to control your alignment and movements.

Action

1 Breathe in as you roll your pelvis backwards, curling your lower spine underneath you and simultaneously curling your head, neck and upper back forwards. The end result should be a lengthened and equally curved spine.

2 Breathe out as you move the pelvis and head simultaneously, unravelling and lengthening your spine back to the Starting Position.

Repeat up to 5 times.

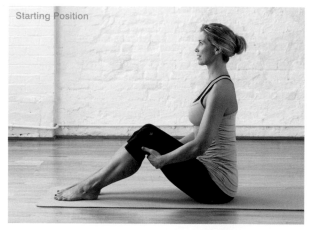

Starting Position

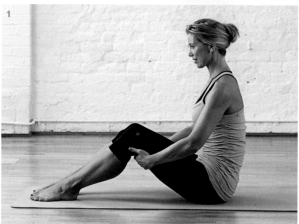

✳
■ Really send the crown of your head up and away from your tailbone. Use your deep abdominal muscles to help to support this C-curve.

■ Aim for an equal amount of flexion throughout the entire length of your spine. Particularly avoid any excessive bending or compression of the neck and head.

■ As you curve over, allow your elbows to bend slightly more, directing them out to the side.

■ Think wide and open across your shoulders, and maintain distance between the ears and the shoulders.

Cat

This is an excellent exercise for developing mobility along the entire length of the spine, while in a position that reduces the pressure on the spine. It teaches you how to control the spine sequentially with both flexion and extension.

✱ Caution: take advice if you have knee problems, and avoid this position if you have recently had a breast operation. ✱

Starting Position

Adopt the Four-point Kneeling Position (p. 32).

Use an appropriate level of core connection to control your alignment and movements.

Action

1 Breathe in and lengthen your spine.

2 Breathe out as you roll your pelvis underneath you, as if directing your tailbone between your legs. As you do so, your lower back will gently round and flex. Continue this flexion and allow your upper back gradually to round, followed by your neck, and finally nod your head slightly forwards. This position is a C-curve (opposite), an even and balanced C shape of the spine.

3 Breathe in, widening the lower ribcage to help maintain this lengthened C-curve.

4 Breathe out as you simultaneously start to unravel the spine from both ends, sending the tailbone away from you, and bringing the pelvis back to neutral as you also lengthen the head and upper spine back to the starting neutral position.

5 Breathe in and maintain the neutral position.

6 Breathe out and shine your breastbone forwards as you gently extend your upper spine. Widen the collarbones.

7 Breathe in and return to the Starting Position.

Repeat up to 10 times.

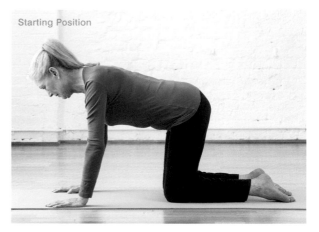

Starting Position

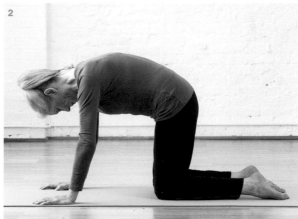

2

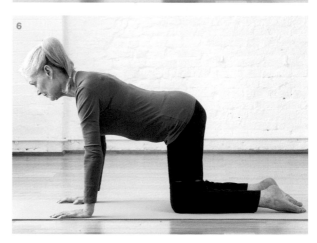

6

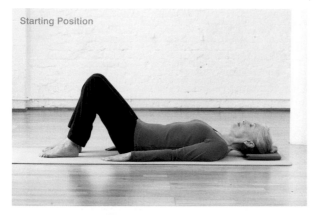

Starting Position

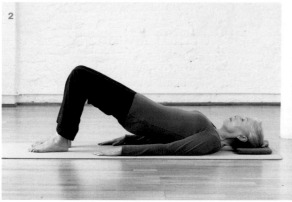

2

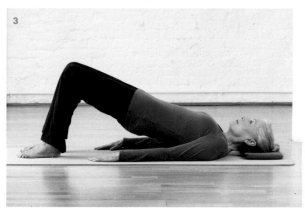

3

Spine Curls

This must be our most popular exercise – you'll find a version of it in nearly every class! Its popularity lies in its ability to gently mobilise your spine by teaching segmental control.

✻ Caution: take advice if you have severe osteoporosis. ✻

Starting Position

The Relaxation Position, arms lengthened down by your sides.

Use an appropriate level of core connection to control your alignment and movements.

Action

1 Breathe in to prepare your body to move.

2 Breathe out as you curl your tailbone under, tilting the pelvis to the north, then peel your spine off the mat one vertebra at a time, lengthening your knees away from your hips. Roll your spine, bone by bone, to the tips of the shoulder blades.

3 Breathe in and hold this position, focusing on the length in your spine.

4 Breathe out as you roll the spine back down, softening the breastbone and wheeling each bone down in turn.

5 Breathe in as you release the pelvis back to level again.

Repeat up to 10 times.

Variation

You could add a Marching feet action at the top of this movement as in Bridge with Marching Feet (p. 95). Note the Watchpoints for this version.

■ Don't roll up too far: maintain a connection of your ribs to your pelvis and avoid arching your spine.

■ Keep equal weight through both feet; this will help to prevent your pelvis dipping to either side.

■ Avoid 'hitching' your pelvis up towards your ribcage; keep the waist equally long on both sides.

■ Keep the knees parallel, in line with your hips, and avoid your feet rolling in or out.

Curl-ups

Like Spine Curls, this is a spinal flexion exercise, but whereas we flexed from the bottom end in Spine Curls, in Curl-ups we flex from the top! This exercise strengthens the abdominal muscles, using them to mobilise the spine and ribcage, while encouraging stability of the pelvis and legs.

✱ Caution: avoid if you have osteoporosis; take advice if you have neck problems. ✱

Starting Position
The Relaxation Position. Lightly clasp both hands behind your head, keeping the elbows open and positioned just in front of your ears, within your peripheral vision.

Use an appropriate level of core connection to control your alignment and movements.

Action
1 Breathe in to prepare.

2 Breathe out as you lengthen the back of your neck and nod your head and sequentially curl up the upper body, keeping the back of your lower ribcage in contact with the mat. Keep your pelvis still and level and do not allow your abdominals to bulge.

3 Breathe in to the back of your ribcage and maintain the curled-up position.

4 Breathe out as you slowly and sequentially roll the spine back down to the mat with control.

Repeat up to 10 times.

✱ ■ Ensure that your pelvis remains grounded in neutral throughout; curl up only as far as you can whilst maintaining this.

■ Although your pelvis remains still, it is essential that the natural curve in your lower spine opens out and releases into the mat; you must not hold this curve.

■ Focus on wheeling your spine off the mat vertebra by vertebra.

■ Control the sequential return of your spine back down to the mat.

■ Focus on your exhalation to encourage your spine to flex forwards and to close your ribcage.

■ Allow your collarbones and shoulder blades to widen, but keep a connection of the shoulder blades to the back ribcage.

■ Allow your head to be heavy and supported in your hands.

■ Keep the neck long and free from tension.

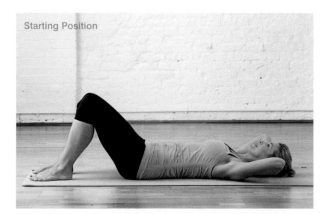

Starting Position

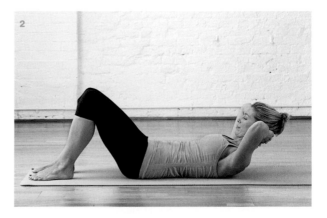

2

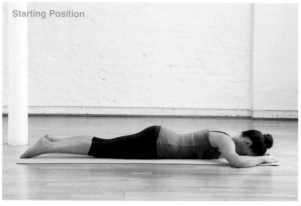

Starting Position

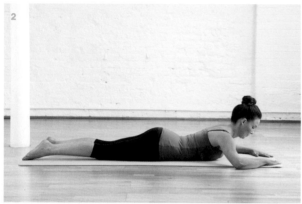

2

SPINAL EXTENSION

This is the opposite movement to spinal flexion. Note that we are talking about thoracic spine extension. These are probably the most important anti-ageing exercises in our programme as they reverse the effects of gravity and help prevent poor posture. They are vital if you have bone-density problems. The watchpoints and caution apply to both exercises.

Diamond Press

This is a great 'first' extension exercise as it teaches you how to move into extension correctly and really targets the upper thoracic area, which is notoriously hard to reach.

Starting Position

Prone. Create a diamond shape with the arms: place the fingertips together, palms down on to the mat and open your elbows. Rest your forehead on the backs of your hands. Alternatively, if it is more comfortable, you may place your hands wider and rest your forehead on a flat cushion. Your legs should be hip-width apart and parallel.

Use an appropriate level of core connection to control your alignment and movements.

✳ Caution: if you have osteoporosis, or if it makes these positions more comfortable, place a folded towel or flat cushion under your abdomen to help support your lower back. Take advice if you have been diagnosed with spinal stenosis – you may prefer to place a small cushion under your waist. ✳

Action

1 Breathe in, preparing your body to move.

2 Breathe out as you lift first your head, then your neck and then your chest off the mat. Feel your lower ribs remaining in contact with the mat, but shine your breastbone forwards, opening your chest.

3 Breathe in as you hold this lengthened and stable position.

4 Breathe out as you lengthen and return your chest, neck and head sequentially back to the Starting Position.

Repeat up to 10 times.

✳ ■ Grow, grow, grow; think forwards and up.

■ Initiate the back extension by lengthening and lifting your head first (think of rolling a marble away along the mat with your nose) and then your neck. When your head and neck are in line with your spine you can start to extend the upper spine.

■ Keep your collarbones wide and open.

■ Keep your lower ribs in contact with the mat as you lift up; this will ensure that you don't lift too far and compress your lower spine. Length through the spine is far more important than height.

■ Avoid putting too much pressure into the arms; they are there to lightly support you.

■ Keep your feet in contact with the mat.

■ As you return back down to the mat, do not collapse; return with length and control.

Cobra Preparation

This helps develop spinal mobility in and around the upper back. Use what you have learned doing the Diamond Press in this exercise.

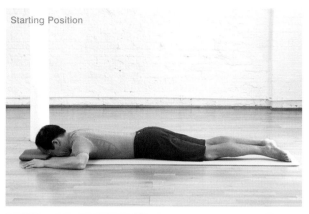

Starting Position

Starting Position

Prone, resting your forehead on the mat. (Use a folded towel if necessary.) Your legs are straight, slightly wider than hip-width, and turned out from the hips. Bend your elbows and position your hands slightly wider than and above your shoulders, your palms facing down. Make sure that your shoulders are released and your collarbones wide.

Use an appropriate level of core connection to control your alignment and movements.

Action

1 Breathe in, preparing your body to move.

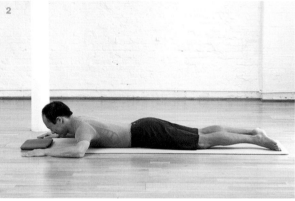

2

2 Breathe out as you begin to lengthen the front of the neck to roll and lift your head and then your chest off the mat. Your arms will begin to straighten slightly. Feel your lower ribs remaining in contact with the mat, but open your chest and focus on directing it forwards.

3 Breathe in as you hold this lengthened and lifted position.

4 Breathe out as you return your chest and head sequentially back down to the mat.

Repeat up to 10 times.

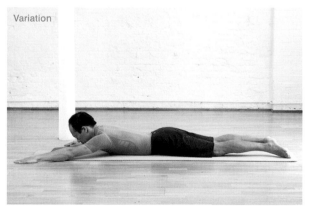

Variation

Variation: Cobra Preparation with One Arm Slide

This challenging variation works on your ability to maintain your upper-back extension and is a great preparation for the exercises on p. 148–55. Be sure to keep your pelvis still.

Follow Action points 1–3 above, then:

4 Breathe out as you slide one arm away along the floor, maintaining your lifted back extension.

5 Breathe in as you slide the arm back to its starting position.

6 Repeat with the other arm, before lengthening and lowering back down to the mat.

✽ Caution: Avoid if you have been diagnosed with stenosis of the spine. ✽

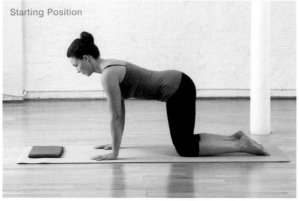

Starting Position

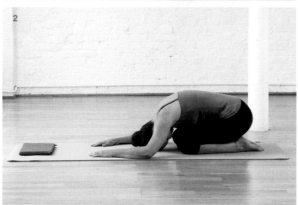

2

Rest Position

We have included Rest Position here in the Fundamentals as it is the natural position/exercise to follow any prone and/or Four-point Kneeling exercises. It is also a great way to encourage lateral breathing, providing an opportunity to refocus concentration in preparation for the next exercise. If you wish, you may also use this position to help pelvic-floor release (p. 177).

Starting Position

From your prone position, come up into Four-point Kneeling.

Action

1 Breathe in, prepare your body, lengthen your spine and bring your feet slightly closer together.

2 Breathe out as you begin to fold at your hips and direct your buttocks backwards and down. Maintain the position of your hands on the mat and lengthen your arms. Ideally, rest your sitting bones on your heels, your chest on your thighs and your forehead on the mat.

3 Breathe in and direct the breath into the back and the sides of your ribs; feel the ribcage progressively expand.

4 Breathe out, fully emptying your lungs, and focus on closing the ribs down and together.

Repeat up to 10 times.

To finish, breathe out and begin by rolling your pelvis underneath you, then sequentially roll and restack your spine to an upright position, sitting back on your heels.

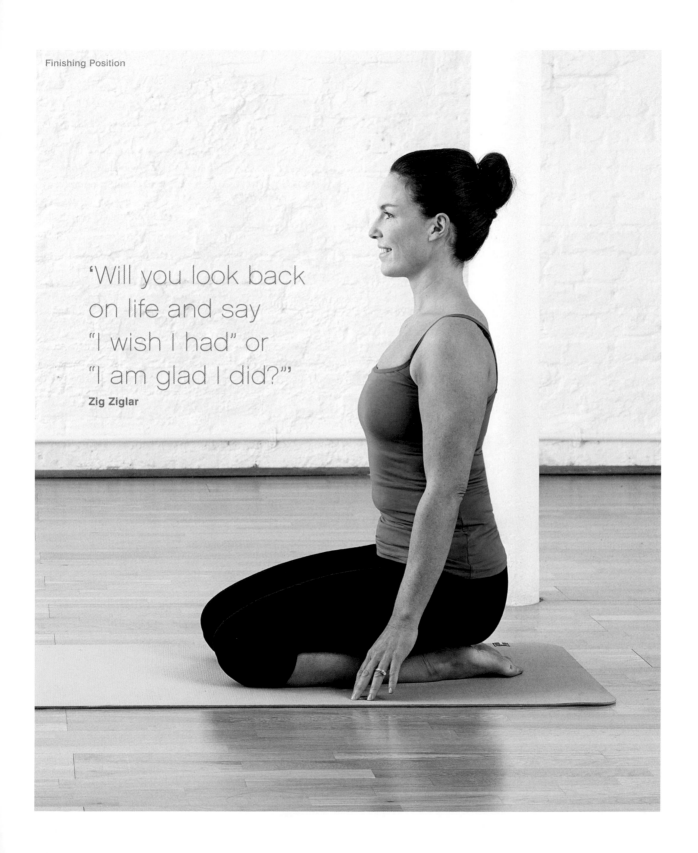

'Will you look back
on life and say
"I wish I had" or
"I am glad I did?"'

Zig Ziglar

SPINAL ROTATION

This movement is vital to the health of the spine as it is one of the first to diminish with old age. All joints love movement and the spine is no exception. Rotation is particularly beneficial as it promotes lubrication.

For most of the rotation exercises we are looking for sequential movement top to bottom or bottom to top. In Waist Twists below, for example, the movement starts with your eyes, as your gaze moves in the direction you are turning, your head follows, then your neck and finally your upper spine. On the way back, the sequence is reversed.

As with all our exercises, lengthening the spine is vital – spiral up, up, up, as you move into the exercise and as you return to the Starting Position.

Waist Twist

This exercise works the muscles around your waist while promoting spinal mobility with a balanced rotation of the head, neck and torso.

Starting Position
This exercise can be performed either seated or standing:

Seated: Sit upright on a chair, with feet hip-width apart on the floor. Fold your arms in front of your chest, just below shoulder height. Place one palm on top of the opposite elbow and the other hand underneath the opposite elbow.

Standing: Stand tall on the floor (not on your mat), legs parallel and hip-width apart. Fold your arms in front of your chest, just below shoulder height, one palm on top of the opposite elbow and the other hand positioned underneath the opposite elbow.

Use an appropriate level of core connection to control your alignment and movements.

Action
1 Breathe in, preparing your body to move, and lengthen your spine.

2 Breathe out as you move your gaze to the right, turning your head, then neck and finally rotating your torso fully to the right. Keep your pelvis still and keep lengthening up through the crown of the head.

3 Breathe in as you continue to lengthen your spine and rotate back to the Starting Position.

Repeat 6 times to each side. After 3 turns, change your arm position so that the underneath arm is now on top.

Variations
■ This exercise can be made easier by folding your arms across your chest.

■ It can be made harder by having your arms stretched out to the sides just below shoulder height and within your peripheral vision.

■ For the most difficult version, lightly clasp your hands behind your neck. Your elbows should be within your peripheral vision. Take care not to pull on the neck.

❋ ■ Your pelvis should remain still. Keep the weight even on either your sitting bones or your feet (depending on your Starting Position) and maintain their contact to the mat/floor throughout.

■ Avoid arching your back or shortening your waist.

■ Carry your arms with the spine; do not allow them to lead the movement.

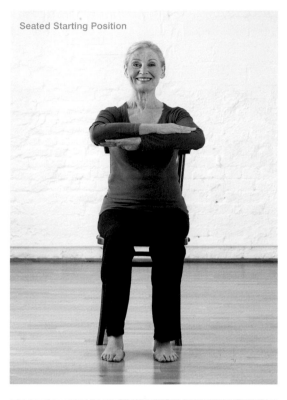

Seated Starting Position

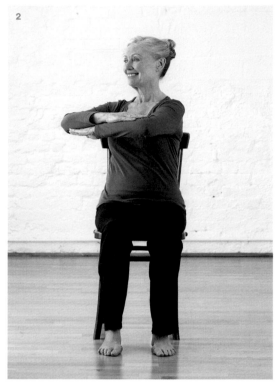

2

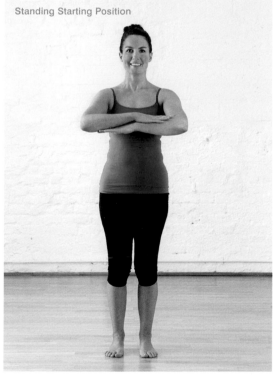

Standing Starting Position

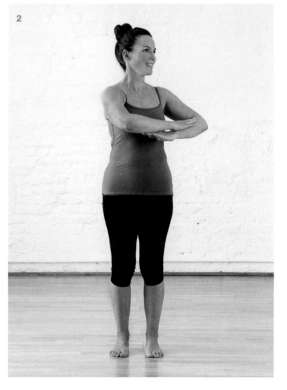

2

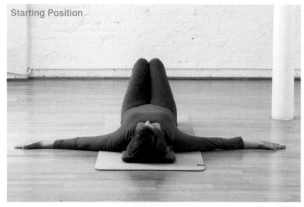

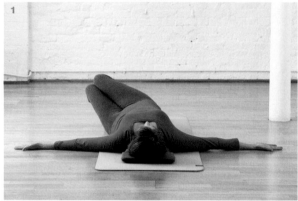

■ Roll your pelvis and your legs directly to the side and avoid any deviation.

■ There should be no shortening on either side of the waist.

■ Maintain a connection between your ribcage and your pelvis and ensure that you don't arch your back as you roll.

■ As you roll, go first through your hips, waist and finally lower ribs, returning lower ribs, waist and finally hips to the mat.

Hip Rolls

The goal here is to challenge your ability to control the sequential rotation of your spine. This exercise also helps to trim your waist!

✱ Caution: take advice if you have back problems. ✱

Starting Position

The Relaxation Position. Bring your legs together and connect your inner thighs. Reach your arms out on the mat slightly lower than shoulder height, palms facing upwards.

Use an appropriate level of core connection to control your alignment and movements.

Action

1 Breathe in and, maintaining the connection of the inner thighs, roll your pelvis to the left (like rolling east in the Compass exercise – p. 24). The right side of the pelvis and the lower right ribs will peel slightly off the mat.

2 Breathe out as you return the pelvis and legs back to the Starting Position, initiating from your centre.

Repeat to the other side, then repeat the whole sequence up to 5 times.

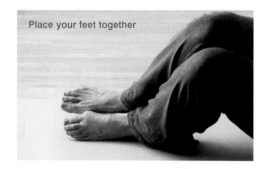

Place your feet together

Bow and Arrow

A feel-good exercise that not only opens your chest, but teaches spinal rotation with control and length.

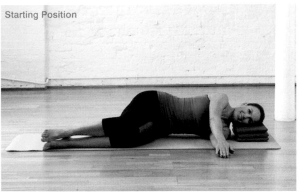

Starting Position

Side-lying on the left, place a substantial cushion (a pillow works fine) underneath your head to ensure that both head and neck are in line with your spine. Bend both knees in front of you so that your hips and knees are bent to a right angle. Place another pillow between your knees as shown in the photo. Lengthen both arms out in front of you at shoulder height, your left arm resting on the mat and your right arm placed on top of it.

Use an appropriate level of core connection to control your alignment and movements.

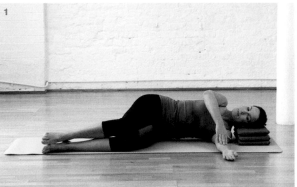

Action

1 Breathe in as you bend your right elbow and slide your hand along the inside of the left arm to the centre of your breastbone. Simultaneously rotate your head, neck and upper spine, but keep your pelvis and spine still.

2 Breathe out as you rotate your spine further to the right, lengthening up through the spine.

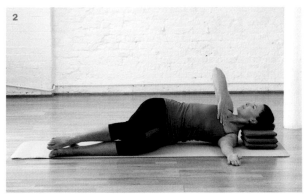

3 Breathe in and straighten your right elbow, lengthening your forearm away from your body. Maintain stillness and stability in your torso.

4 Breathe out as you rotate, lengthen and return your spine to the Starting Position. Keep your right arm straight and move from the shoulder joint to come back to the Starting Position.

Repeat up to 5 times, then repeat on the other side.

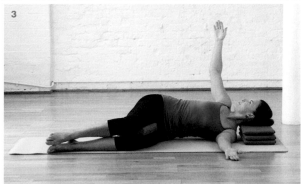

Bow and Arrow – Sitting and High Kneeling

The upright position used here is more challenging than the version on p. 67. You have a choice of Starting positions – High Kneeling offers the biggest challenge.

✻ Caution: take advice if you have back problems. ✻

Starting Position

Either: Sit tall on a sturdy chair with your feet hip-width apart and parallel, or sit on the mat with knees bent and the soles of your feet together. The feet should be quite a distance from the body to allow a feeling of space in the hip joints. You may sit on a cushion if it helps.
Or: Use a High Kneeling starting position.

Your arms should be lengthened in front of you, slightly lower than shoulder height and shoulder-width apart; they should be parallel, palms facing down.

Use an appropriate level of core connection to control your alignment and movements.

Action

1 Breathe in to prepare.

2 Breathe out as you bend your left elbow, drawing the arm towards your body and your left hand towards the shoulder. Simultaneously rotate your head, neck and upper spine (in that order) to the left.

3 Breathe in as you straighten the arm while lengthening the spine and encouraging a little more rotation.

4 Breathe out as you rotate your spine back to the Starting Position, keeping the arm straight.

5 Repeat 5 times on each side.

> ✳ ■ Keep spiralling up, up, up as you turn.
> ■ Ensure that your pelvis remains stable.
> ■ Avoid arching your back or bending to the side.

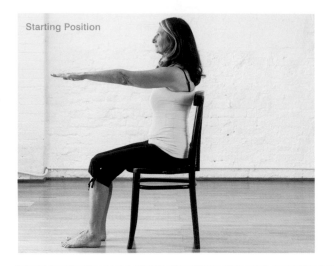
Starting Position

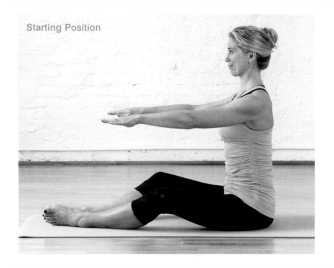
Starting Position

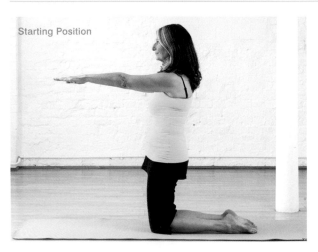
Starting Position

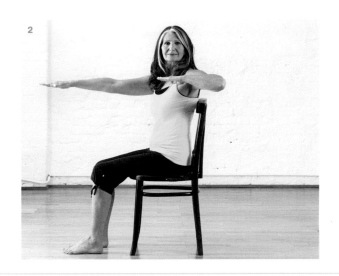

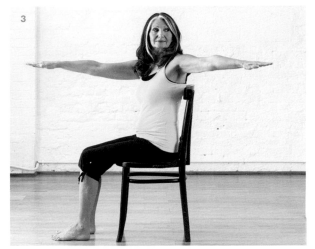

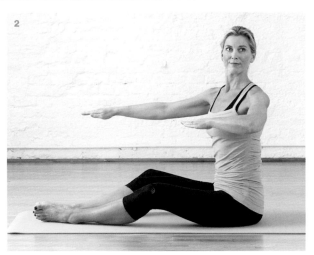

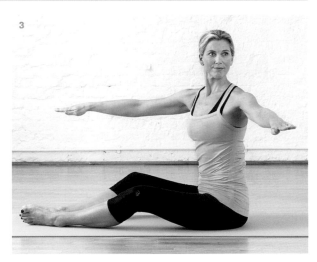

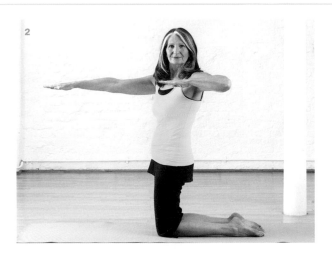

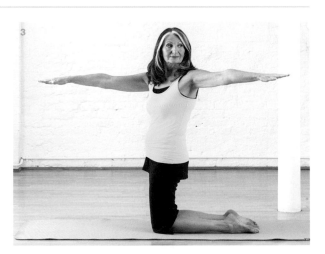

SPINAL LATERAL FLEXION

As you bend to the side, your spine moves into lateral flexion. Ideally, we want to encourage sequential lateral flexion and spinal length. As you reach over, initiate the movement with an incline of your head and continue moving through your neck and then your ribcage. Reverse the sequence as you return to the upright position, always maintaining length in your spine and focusing on the connection to your centre.

Side Reach

This exercise teaches you to lengthen out as you mobilise your spine in lateral flexion. It is a real feel-good exercise, enabling you to stretch out your spine and sides. As with Hip Rolls (p. 66), it has the added benefit of trimming the waist. Once again, you have a choice of starting positions.

Starting Position
Either: Stand tall on the floor (not on your mat) and lengthen your spine into neutral. Your legs are parallel, but slightly wider than hip-width apart. Allow your arms to lengthen down by your sides.

Or: Sit tall with your legs bent and turned out, and the soles of your feet connected. Your feet should be quite a distance from the body to allow a feeling of space in the hip joints with your pelvis and spine in neutral. Allow your arms to lengthen down by your sides. If you find it difficult to sit with a neutral pelvis and spine in this position, sit on a cushion or rolled-up towel to help attain the correct alignment. (This exercise may also be performed seated on a chair; feet placed hip-width apart on the floor.)

Or: High Kneel.

Use an appropriate level of core connection to control your alignment and movements.

Starting Position

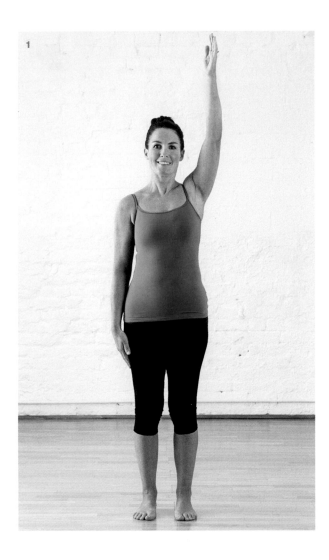

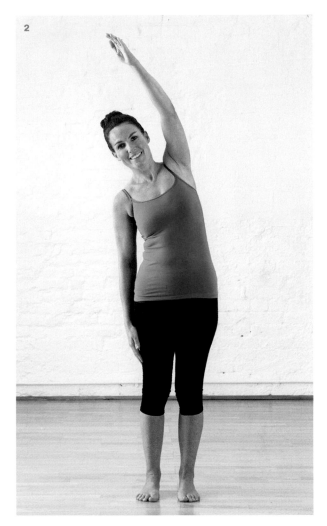

Action

1 Breathe in as you raise your left arm out to the side and overhead, as in Floating Arms (p. 52).

2 Breathe out as you reach up and over and, leading with your head, sequentially bend your spine to the right. Maintain the relationship between the left arm and your head. If sitting, your right arm will reactively slide further along the mat and then bend, so that your forearm can support your position. If standing or High Kneeling, your right arm will remain lengthened and slide down the outside of your right leg.

3 Breathe in. Maintain the length and position of your spine and focus on breathing laterally.

4 Breathe out as you return the spine back to the vertical position. Lower your left arm down by your side.

Repeat 5 times on each side.

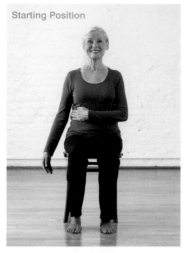

Starting Position

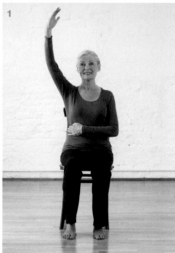

1

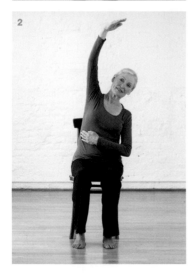

2

Variation: Side Reach with Breathing

In this version you will be working on the mobility of your ribs and your breathing technique. It is particularly helpful if you have any respiratory problems.

Starting Position

As on p. 70, but place your left hand on the right side of the ribcage.

Use an appropriate level of core connection to control your alignment and movements.

Action

Follow Action Points 1 and 2 on p. 71, this time raising your right arm. Your left hand stays on your ribs.

3 Breathe in, allowing the left side to expand into your hand.

4 Breathe out as you return to the Starting Position, allowing the ribs to release and gently pulling with the right hand.

Repeat 5 times on each side.

- Think of length in both sides of the waist to avoid compression.

- Ensure that you move in one plane only, directly to the side.

- Maintain openness across your chest and the back of your shoulders, avoiding overreaching with your arms.

- Keep your head and neck in line with the rest of your spine.

COMBINED MOVEMENTS

The exercises so far have demonstrated the spine moving into pure flexion, extension, rotation and lateral flexion. You will need to learn how to do these movements slowly with control. Once this is mastered, you can start exercises which have combined movements, for example Oblique Curls (below) which involve flexion and rotation of the spine. Many of the exercises in the Main Programme mirror the complex integrated movements of our everyday activities.

Oblique Curl-ups

Similar to Curl Ups (p. 59), this exercise strengthens the abdominals, using them to mobilise the spine and ribcage. The addition of rotation to the curling movement adds another dimension of challenge, particularly when maintaining the stability of the pelvis and legs.

✳ Caution: avoid if you have osteoporosis and take advice if you have neck problems. ✳

Starting Position
The Relaxation Position. Lightly clasp both hands behind your head, keeping the elbows open and positioned just in front of your ears, within your peripheral vision.

Use an appropriate level of core connection to control your alignment and movements.

Action
1 Breathe in, preparing your body to move.

2 Breathe out as you nod your head and sequentially curl up the upper body, rotating your head and torso to the left and directing the right side of your ribcage towards your left hip. Keep your pelvis still and level and do not allow your abdominals to bulge.

3 Breathe into the back of your ribcage and maintain the curled and rotated position.

4 Breathe out as you slowly and sequentially roll back down to the centre with control.

5 Repeat, this time rotating to the right.

Repeat up to 10 times.

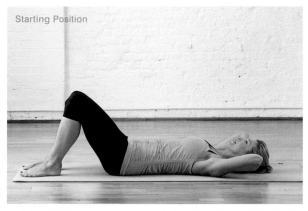
Starting Position

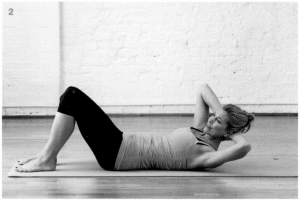
2

✳ ■ Ensure that your pelvis remains grounded in neutral and square throughout; curl up only as far you can whilst maintaining this.

■ Focus on wheeling and rotating your spine off the mat, vertebra by vertebra.

■ The rotation should come from the movement of the ribs on the spine and the spine itself. Try not to pull on your head and neck.

■ Keep both sides of your waist equally long.

■ Allow your head to be heavy and supported in your hands; rotate it in relation to the rotation in your spine – no more and no less.

OTHER FUNDAMENTAL SKILLS

Hip Hinge

The ability to bend from the hips with a 'straight' spine is an essential movement skill to master as you age if you wish to avoid constantly bending from the waist. This is a priority if you have osteoporosis. It will also help you with the Pilates Squat (opposite). The movement should come from the hips, not the spine, which should stay lengthened and move as one. Sounds strange, but imagine that you have swallowed a long stick!

Starting Position

Sit tall on a sturdy chair, feet hip-width apart and parallel. You will need to be nearer the edge than the back of the chair. Place your hands palms down in the crease where your legs meet your pelvis.

Use an appropriate level of core connection to control your alignment and movements.

Action

1 Breathe in to prepare to move.

2 Breathe out and, keeping the spine straight (but with its natural curves), hinge forwards from this crease. The spine should move as one long unit.

3 Breathe in as you hinge back to upright. Repeat up to 5 times.

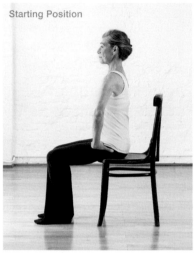

Starting Position

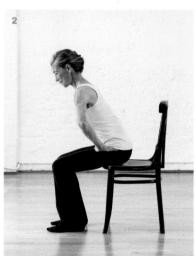

2

■ Take care not to tip your head back. The back of the neck should remain lengthened.

■ Check that you are moving solely from the hips.

■ Keep lengthening through the spine, at the top and bottom ends!

Pilates Squat and Hinge

Practise the Hip Hinge (opposite) before trying this exercise, which works on many levels to strengthen and mobilise your hips and lower limbs.

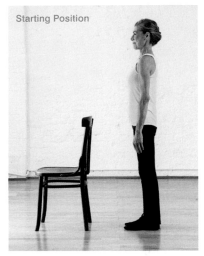

Starting Position

Initially, practise this standing sideways to a wall or in front of a sturdy chair, in case you lose your balance. Once again, imagine you have swallowed a long stick. Stand tall, arms relaxed down by your side, palms facing inwards.

Use an appropriate level of core connection to control your alignment and movements.

Action

1 Breathe in to prepare the body; lengthen through the spine as you bend the knees and the hips simultaneously to hinge forwards slightly from the hips.

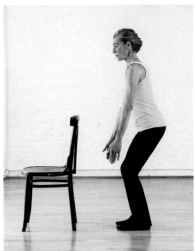

2 As you do so, reach forwards with both arms – it will help to counter your balance.

3 Breathe out as you straighten the legs and return to the upright Starting Position.

Repeat up to 10 times.

Variation

Try this exercise holding light weights in each hand.

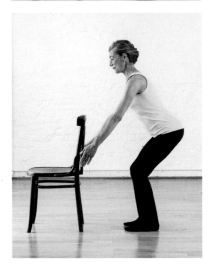

* ■ This is a small squat, so do not go down too far and avoid lowering the pelvis below knee level.

■ Check that your ankles, knees and hips are lined up as you hinge forward.

■ Do not allow your knees or ankles to buckle in or out.

■ As you straighten up, press the floor away evenly through the soles of the feet.

■ Keep the heels in contact with the floor throughout.

■ Sense the spine lengthening up and away.

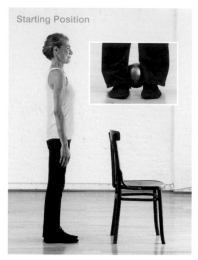

Starting Position

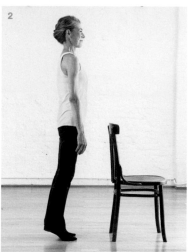

2

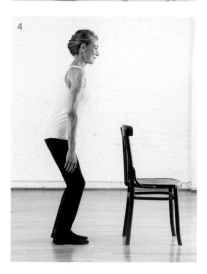

4

Tennis Ball Rising

This involves a similar movement to the Pilates Squat (p. 75), but has more elements. It helps connect and centre your body with your legs, while mobilising and strengthening the ankles and feet. It also helps develop balance and control. You will need a small ball.

Starting Position

Stand tall on the floor (not on your mat) and lengthen your spine into neutral. Your legs are parallel and slightly closer than hip-width apart; place a tennis (or similar-sized) ball in between your ankles, just below the inside ankle bones. If necessary, have a sturdy chair slightly in front of you in case you need it for balance.

Use an appropriate level of core connection to control your alignment and movements.

Action

1 Breathe in, preparing to move, and lengthen your spine.

2 Breathe out and rise up on to the balls of your feet, lifting your heels off the floor. Keep your spine lengthened and stable and maintain the position of the ball.

3 Breathe in as you lower your heels back down to the floor with control and maintaining length on the spine.

4 Breathe out as you softly bend your knees, keeping your heels firmly pressing into the floor.

5 Breathe in as you straighten your legs and return to the Starting Position. Repeat up to 10 times.

■ Remain long in your waist, maintain a stable pelvis and keep a sense of your spine lengthening up and away.

■ Keep your weight balanced evenly on both feet. Also, do not allow your feet to roll either in or out.

■ Fully lengthen your legs, but don't lock your knees.

■ Maintain correct alignment of your legs; ensure your ankles and knees remain in line with your hips.

Thumb Rolls

Here, the skill is to roll the humerus (upper-arm bone) in the shoulder joint socket without rolling your shoulders forwards and back.

* Caution: Take advice if you have a shoulder problem *

Starting Position

This exercise may be done standing or sitting tall on a sturdy chair (one without arms). Place your right hand on your upper left shoulder (to check for any unwanted movement). Your left arm should be lengthened down by your side, palm facing inwards and left thumb lifted out a little (as if you are going to hitch a lift). Your collarbones should be wide and open.

Use an appropriate level of core connection to control your alignment and movements.

Action

1 Breathe in and prepare for movement.

2 Breathe out as you roll the thumb, accompanied by the whole arm, outwards. Keep the shoulder still, do not allow it to roll back.

3 Breathe in as you roll the thumb and arm back inwards, taking care not to roll the shoulder inwards.

Repeat up to 8 times, then repeat with the other arm.

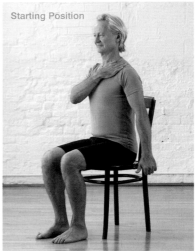

Starting Position

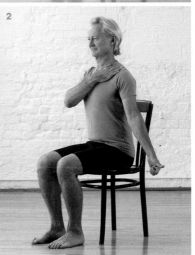

2

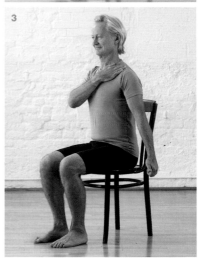

3

* ■ Keep your collarbones wide and open.

■ The thumb should be used to guide the movement.

■ Keep the working arm straight but take care not to hyperextend the elbow (that is, do not lock it out).

■ Keep lengthening up through the spine.

■ Keep your focus forwards and soft.

VISUAL SKILLS

When we said that no part of the body was going to be ignored, we meant it!

We have already mentioned that vision is affected by the ageing process. The exercises in this section have been designed to improve your visual skills and work in a number of different ways.

Training and conditioning the visual system means working the muscles associated with eye movements and eye–body reflexes, enabling us to quickly and accurately recognise and process visual information and to improve:

■ field vision and peripheral awareness
■ mental visualisation
■ reaction time and anticipation
■ attention, focus and concentration
■ balance, speed and agility.

Visual skills can be divided into two groups: visual motor skills, which generally relate to our ability to move and adjust the eyes; and visual perceptual skills, which relate to our visual memory and visual sequential memory, having more to do with our ability to process visual information.

'Do things that make you happy, with people who make you happy, and be happy with the person you are now.' Leo Babauta

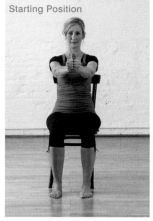
Starting Position
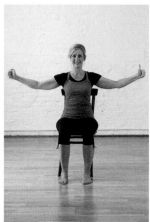

Peripheral Vision/Awareness Exercise
Peripheral vision is the body's first way of sending messages of movement to the brain; it is essential to improving anticipation and reaction speed.

Starting Position
Stand tall or sit on a sturdy chair. Have your arms stretched out in front, thumbs together and facing up. Keep your gaze focused and still between your thumbs.

Action
Your eyes look forwards throughout the exercise. Spread your thumbs out; once you reach the limit of your vision field, wiggle your thumbs.

Return to the Starting Position and repeat with no strain.

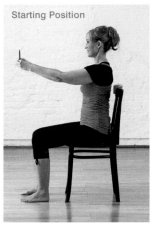
Starting Position

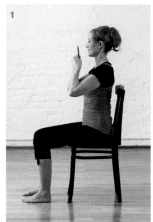
1

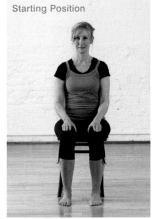
Starting Position

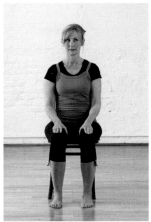

Pencil Exercise

This exercise helps to train perception, alignment and spatial localisation skills, as well as conditioning the eye muscles.

Starting Position

Sit tall on a sturdy chair with your arms straight out at shoulder level. Hold a pencil vertically.

Action

1 With eyes focused on the tip of the pencil, slowly bring the pencil towards your nose while continuing to focus on the pencil tip.

2 As the pencil nears your nose, you will see two pencils instead of one. At this point of double vision, hold the pencil still and focus on it for 10 seconds.

3 Then slowly return the pencil to its original position at arm's length.

Repeat this process for 60 seconds.

Spotlight Exercise

Starting Position

Sit tall on a chair, looking forwards.

Action

Imagine a moving spotlight on the wall in front of you and, without moving your head, follow the spotlight side to side, right-left-right, left-right-left, up-down, up-right, up-left, down-right, down-left, moving inwards and outwards.

Repeat with no strain.

Contrast Sensitivity

This exercise helps our ability to identify objects quickly and clearly in different lighting conditions and against backgrounds of varying colour.

Starting Position

Sit or stand tall, looking at a small object which is either on the floor, on a table or at eye level.

Action

Look through the object and focus on somewhere darker far away, then adjust your focus back to the object. Repeat the above with the object in a brighter light.

Repeat with no strain.

Eye–Hand Co-ordination: Shape the Hand

Eye–hand exercises like this are great for improving your ability to synchronise finger, hand and arm movements with constantly changing visual information, thus improving your timing and reaction speed.

Starting Position
Sit tall about 30cm from a table on which there are objects varying in size and shape.

Action
Choose one object and look at it for some seconds. Then look at the other objects and decide on one of them to pick up. Before you pick it up it, look at the shape of your hand. It should have formed itself into the shape of the chosen object.

Repeat the above with all the objects placed on the table in turn.

Variation
You may repeat the above in a standing position or while walking.

Eye–Foot Co-ordination: Drills and Turn the Head

These exercises help your ability to synchronise foot, knee and leg movements with constantly changing visual information. Eye–foot co-ordination refers to our ability to quickly and efficiently change direction. This is advantageous when walking over unpredictable terrain, when we may be required to react quickly without losing our balance.

Starting Position for Drills
Stand tall with your feet hip-width apart and arms down by your sides. Keep your head still while moving your eyes.

Action
1 Look to the right with your eyes, keeping your head still. Step to the right with the right foot followed by the left.

2 Bring your feet together.

3 Repeat, stepping to the left.

4 Repeat the sequence moving forwards.

5 Repeat the above, moving backwards.

Variation
Take one step forward and, once back in the Starting Position, take one step back. You may do two steps forwards and two back.

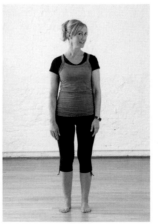
Turn the Head

Starting Position for Turn the Head
Stand tall.

Action
Walk in a straight line, turning the head and eyes alternately right and left; keep walking in the same direction.

Then, keeping your gaze fixed on an object, walk changing direction, moving right, left and diagonally.

Starting Position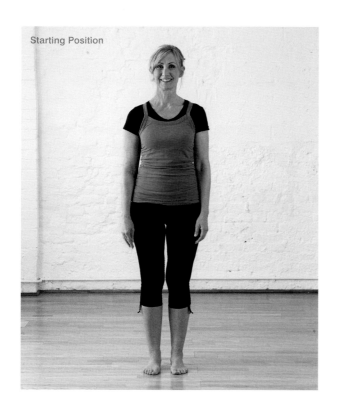

1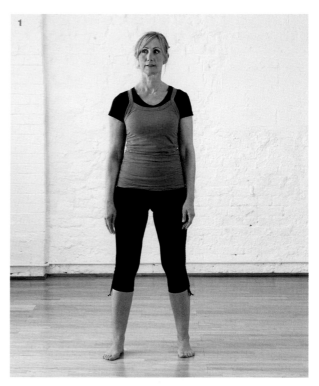

2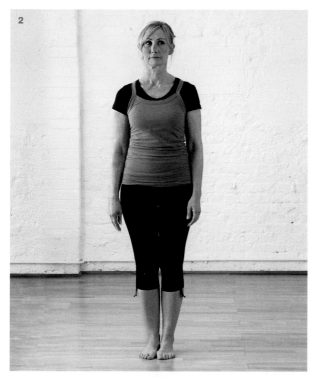

4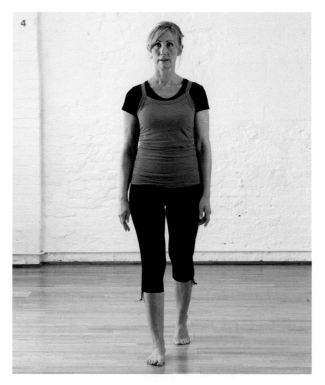

FUNDAMENTAL WORKOUTS

Here are some suggestions for three balanced workouts of about 45 minutes in length.

You can create your own workouts, too. Start each workout with exercises which gently mobilise your joints (such as Starfish and Spine Curls). Include all the spinal movements of flexion, extension, rotation and side flexion (unless you have been advised against one of them). Balance upper and lower body. Try to finish with a standing exercise. And remember that even a 15 minute workout will make a difference!

Workout One

- Starting Position: Relaxation Position (p. 23)
- Compass (p. 24)
- Chin Tucks and Neck Rolls (p. 26)
- Shoulder Drops (p. 46)
- Ribcage Closure (p. 47)
- Knee Openings (pp. 42–43)
- Spine Curls (p. 58)
- Curl-ups (p. 59)
- Hip Rolls (p. 66)
- Oyster (p. 51)
- Diamond Press (p. 60)
- Star Preparation (p. 49)
- Cat (p. 57)
- Rest Position (p. 62)
- Seated Bow and Arrow (p. 68–9)
- Scarf Breathing (p. 36)
- A vision exercise (pp. 78–81)
- Hip Hinge (p. 74)
- Standing Side Reach (pp. 70-1)
- Standing on One Leg (p. 53)
- Pilates Squat (p. 75)

Workout Two

- Starting Position: Standing (p. 34)
- Floating Arms (p. 52)
- Waist Twist (p. 64)
- Relaxation Position (p. 23)
- Compass (p. 24)
- Single Knee Folds (pp. 44)
- Knee Openings (pp. 42–43)
- Starfish (p. 48)
- Spine Curls (p. 58)
- Oblique Curl-ups (p. 73)
- Cobra Preparation (p. 61)
- Prone Knee Lifts (p. 49)
- Table Top Preparation (p. 50)
- Rest Position (p. 62)
- Scarf Breathing (p. 36)
- The Wind Zip (p. 40)
- Side Reach with Breathing (p. 72)
- A vision exercise (pp. 78–81)
- Seated C-Curve (p. 56)
- Side-lying Bow and Arrow (p. 67)
- Tennis Ball Rising (p. 76)
- Pilates Squat (p. 75)

Workout Three

- Starting Position: Seated on a Chair (p. 28)
- Hand Press (p. 29)
- Scarf Breathing (p. 36)
- The Nod (p. 27)
- Thumb Rolls (p. 77)
- Seated Bow and Arrow (p. 68–9)
- Hip Hinge (p. 74)
- Relaxation position (p. 23)
- Shoulder Drops (p. 46)
- Ribcage Closure (p. 47)
- Leg Slides (pp. 42–43)
- Spine curls (p. 58)
- Curl-ups (p. 59)
- Hip Rolls (p. 66)
- Diamond Press (p. 60)
- Prone Knee Lifts (p. 49)
- Cat (p. 57)
- Rest Position (p. 62)
- Oyster (p. 51)
- Standing on One Leg (p. 53)
- Waist Twist (p. 64)
- Tennis Ball Rising (p. 76)

MAIN EXERCISE PROGRAMME

The following exercises may be used alongside the Fundamentals to create balanced workouts. If you have a medical condition, please refer to the appropriate chapters for advice.

Remember to alternate the leg, arm, direction or side you start with each time you work out. And remember, the stated number of repetitions is a guideline only – it's quality of movement, not quantity, which counts.

For some suggested workouts, see pp. 142–43.

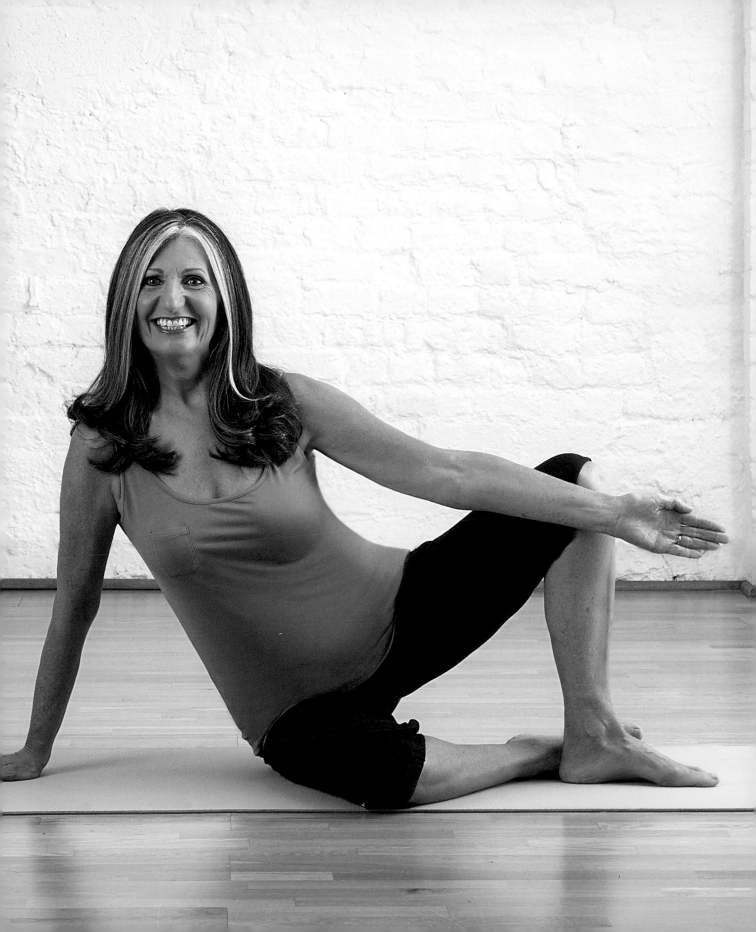

MAIN EXERCISE PROGRAMME

Knee Rolls

An important exercise for mobilising the hips, this also teaches you to move your legs independently from your pelvis. This skill is equally important for the health of your back. The action should come from the top of the thigh bones rolling in the hip socket.

✳ Caution: take advice/avoid if you have had a recent hip replacement (that is, in the last three months). ✳

Starting Position

The Relaxation Position, but place your feet slightly wider than hip-width apart. Have your arms out on the mat slightly lower than shoulder height with your palms facing down (see below for a progression).

Use an appropriate level of core connection to control your alignment and movements.

Action

1 Breathe in, preparing your body to move.

2 Breathe out as you roll your left leg in and your right leg out, both moving from the hip joint. (Both knees will therefore roll to the left.) Allow your feet to peel slightly off the mat.

3 Breathe out and return both legs to the centre at the same time.

4 Repeat the roll on the other side and then repeat the whole sequence up to 5 times.

Variation

Try Knee Rolls as above, but with the arms up in the Starting Position for Shoulder Drops (p. 46). This offers a greater challenge to your stability.

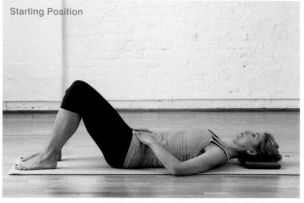

Starting Position

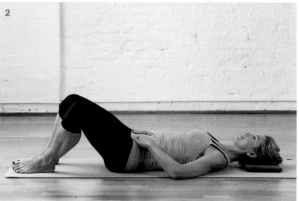

2

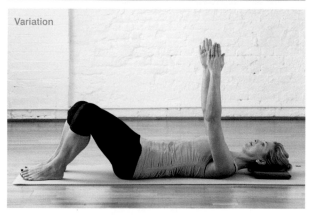

Variation

✱ ■ Keep your pelvis as still and square as possible. Your pelvis will want to roll with your legs, and your goal is to stop it, but there will some movement. Imagine a magnet connecting the inner thighs – try to keep the same distance between the thighs as your legs roll.

Variation: Prone Knee Rolls

This exercise may also be done lying in a prone position. As before, the goal is to mobilise your hips. This version makes it easier to keep your pelvis still, so you get a sense of where you are moving from – your hip joint.

✳ Caution: take advice if you have had a hip replacement in the last 6–12 weeks. ✳

Starting Position

Lie prone with your forehead resting on your folded hands or use a pillow if that feels more comfortable. Have your legs slightly wider than hip-width apart and bend one knee.

Use an appropriate level of core connection to control your alignment and movements.

Action

1 Breathe in, to prepare to move.

2 Breathe out as you roll the bent knee inwards, moving the thigh bone from the hip joint.

3 Breathe in and roll the thigh bone back to the Starting Position, but do not stop there...

4... breathe out as you continue to roll the leg outwards.

5 Breathe in as you bring your leg back to the Starting Position.

Repeat up to 5 times with each leg.

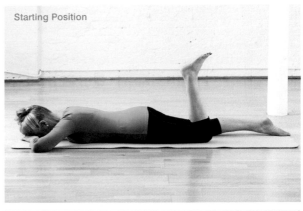
Starting Position

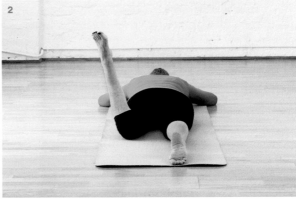
2

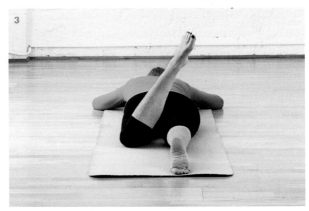
3

■ Stay in control of the movement; do not allow your leg to fall away from you.

■ The knee of the moving leg stays bent.

■ Your pelvis stays remains still and centred.

Zig-zags

This exercise has the same goal as Knee Rolls (p. 86) – to mobilise the hip joint. It can be done in a variety of ways and positions. In this version we are working with one leg at a time in the Relaxation Position. You will need to be able to slide your leg freely. If your floor surface is not suitable, you can place your foot on a piece of paper so that it slides.

✻ Caution: take advice regarding the inward rotation (Actions 3 and 4) of the thigh movement if you have had a hip replacement in the last 6–12 weeks. You may still be able to do the exercise, but bring the leg back in a parallel position rather than turning the thigh in. ✻

Starting Position
The Relaxation Position, but with your left leg stretched out along the mat in line with your hip. Check that your pelvis is still in neutral.

Use an appropriate level of core connection to control your alignment and movements.

Action
1 Breathe in to prepare, and open your right knee, keeping your pelvis stable (as for Knee Openings, p. 43).

2 Breathe out as you slide the right leg away, keeping the heel of your foot in line with your hip joint.

3 Breathe in as you turn the whole leg inwards from the hip, keeping the pelvis still.

4 Breathe out as you bend the knee and draw the leg back up once again, keeping the heel in line with your hip. Maintain the internal rotation of the leg for as long as possible.

5 Breathe in as you turn out the thigh in the hip joint again.

6 Breathe out as you slide the leg away.

Repeat this action 3 times, then reverse the movement by turning in at the hip to begin. Repeat the sequence with the left leg.

■ Try to keep your pelvis as still and stable as possible, especially as you roll the thigh bone in and out.

■ Remember where your hip joints are and do not let the leg wander off to the side.

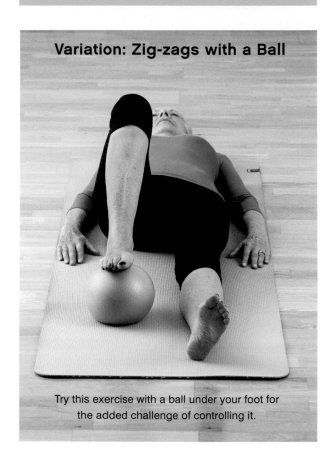

Variation: Zig-zags with a Ball

Try this exercise with a ball under your foot for the added challenge of controlling it.

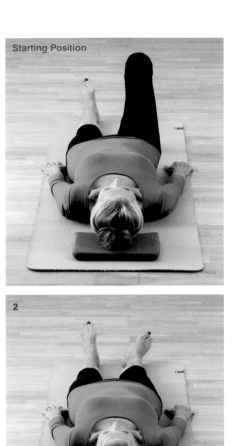

Starting Position

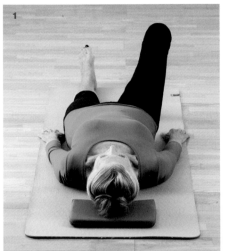

1

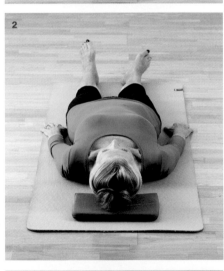

2

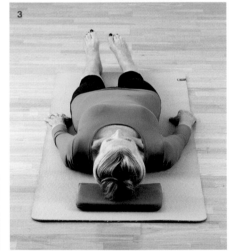

3

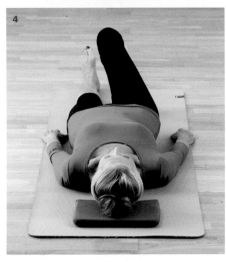

4

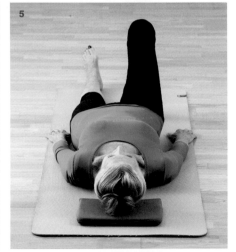

5

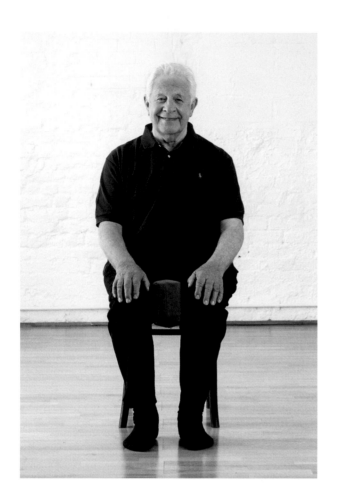

Seated Pillow Squeeze

Even though you are seated for this exercise, it is very useful in preventing falls as it helps to strengthen your inner-thigh muscles, while challenging your ability to keep good posture.

Starting Position

Sit tall on a sturdy chair, feet and knees hip-width apart and parallel (place your feet on a few books/ a step if you are short in the leg!). Place a pillow between your knees. Check that your weight is evenly distributed.

Use an appropriate level of core connection to control your alignment and movements.

Action

1 Breathe in to prepare.

2 Breathe out as you gently squeeze the pillow between your knees without losing any height. Keep your pelvis and spine in neutral.

3 Breathe in and release the pillow.

Repeat up to 10 times.

'Old age can be ... a growing into ourselves. We are still the same people who we always have been, but we are more deeply so.'
Molly Andrews, 'The Seductiveness of Agelessness'

■ As you squeeze, check that no unwanted tension creeps in elsewhere in the body.

■ Keep shoulders open and collarbones wide.

Windows

This is great to help you organise your shoulders and open out the front of your chest.

✳ Caution: take advice if you have a shoulder problem. ✳

Starting Position
The Relaxation Position. Lift both arms vertically above your chest, shoulder-width apart, as for Shoulder Drops on p. 46 but with your palms facing forwards.

Use an appropriate level of core connection to control your alignment and movements.

Action
1 Breathe in to prepare.

2 Breathe out as you bend both elbows, directing them down towards the mat and in line with your shoulders.

3 Breathe in as you rotate the arms, lowering the forearms and the backs of your hands back towards the mat.

4 Breathe out as you straighten the arms, reaching them overhead as in Ribcage Closure (p. 47).

5 Breathe in as you straighten the arms back up to the Starting Position.

Repeat up to 5 times.

Variation: Reverse Windows
In this variation you reverse the Windows arm action. Feel the muscles deep underneath your shoulders helping to draw the arms down as your upper shoulders stay relaxed and open.

Action
Follow Actions 1–4 above, then:

5 Breathe in as you maintain the Ribcage Closure position.

6 Breathe out as you draw the arms back down alongside your shoulders. Take care not to draw them down too far.

7 Breathe in as you rotate the arms back into the Action 2 position; you are ready then to follow Action Point 3.

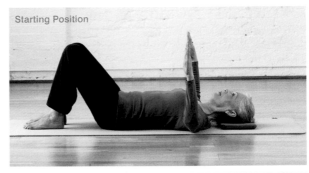
Starting Position

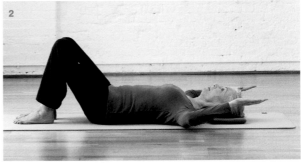
2

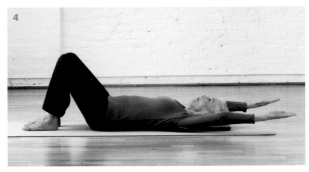
4

■ Remember what you learned in Ribcage Closure on p. 47.

■ Your elbows may not reach the mat, depending on your flexibility. Do not force the movement.

■ Keep your pelvis and spine stable and still.

■ Try to keep your forearm and upper arm on the same plane when straightening the arms.

■ Try to keep good alignment at the wrists; do not bend them, keep them in line with your hands and elbows.

■ Keep your neck long and free from tension.

Arm Circles

Great for mobilising the shoulders and freeing up any hidden tension in this area. Study the photos closely to see how the arms rotate in the shoulder sockets as they move through the circle. You have a choice of Starting Positions – standing will be most challenging. Note the changes to palm/arm position.

* Caution: take advice if you have a shoulder injury. *

Starting Position
Either: The Relaxation Position, lengthening your arms by your sides, palms facing downwards.

Or: Sitting tall in a chair, palms facing backwards.

Or: Standing tall, palms facing backwards.

Use an appropriate level of core connection to control your alignment and movements.

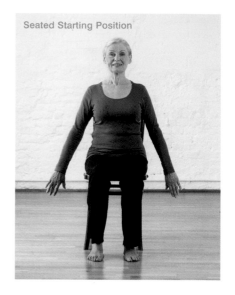
Seated Starting Position

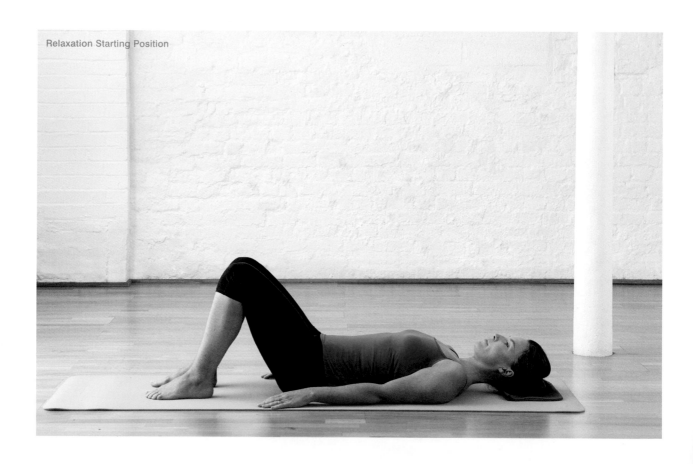
Relaxation Starting Position

Action

1 Breathe in, preparing your body to move.

2 Breathe out as you raise both arms above the chest, and then reach them overhead. Focus on softly closing down the ribcage as you exhale.

3 Breathe in as you circle your arms out to the side and down towards the body, palms facing up if you are in the Relaxation position, forwards if you are sitting or standing. Just before your arms return to the Starting Position, turn your palms downwards if you are in Relaxation Position, or backwards if you are sitting or standing.

Repeat up to 5 times, then reverse the direction.

■ If you are standing, make sure that your arms circle slightly in front of you, within your peripheral vision.

■ Remember what you learned in Ribcage Closure and Floating Arms (pp. 47 and 52). As the arms circle back down, lead with your little fingers.

■ Allow your shoulder blades to glide freely on the back of your ribcage, but maintain the distance between your ears and shoulders.

■ Fully lengthen your arms, but avoid locking your elbows.

■ Keep your neck long and free from tension.

■ Keep your pelvis and spine stable and still throughout. Be particularly careful not to allow your upper spine to arch as you reach your arms overhead.

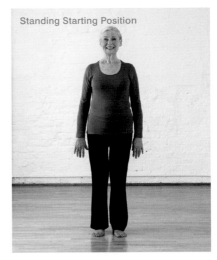

Standing Starting Position

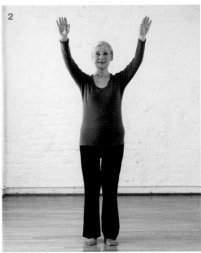

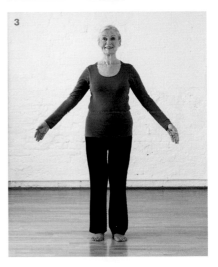

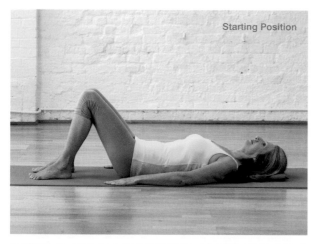
Starting Position

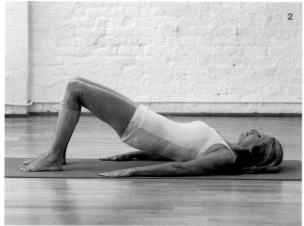
2

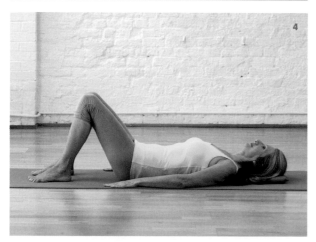
4

Bridge

There is absolutely no way we are letting you get flabby buttocks! We cannot stress enough how important it is to have tone in the gluteals, especially as you age, and there will be several variations of this great exercise throughout the book.

✱ Caution: Take advice if you are recovering from a knee operation ✱

Starting Position

The Relaxation Position. It's preferable not to have a pillow or towel under your head, but your head should be in line with your neck, so if you need one it is OK. You may also place a small cushion between your thighs if you wish.

Use an appropriate level of core connection to control your alignment and movements.

Action

1 Breathe in to prepare your body to move.

2 Breathe out as you send your knees away from you and lift your bottom up from the mat, raising your spine in one movement until you end up in a long diagonal line.

3 Breathe in and hold the position.

4 Breathe out and lower the spine in one piece.

Repeat up to 10 times.

■ Do not be tempted to curl the spine; it moves as one (imagine you have swallowed a long stick).

■ If you use a cushion, do not squeeze it – use it to help you maintain your alignment.

■ If you find the backs of your thighs going into spasm as you lift, focus on your gluteals more.

Variation: Bridge with Marching Feet

In this version you add the action of marching feet at the height of the Bridge. This adds the extra challenge of controlling weight transfer. For perfect marching feet try the exercise on p. 134.

Starting Position

As opposite.

Use an appropriate level of core connection to control your alignment and movements.

Action

Follow Action points 1 and 2 opposite, then:

3 Breathe in as you lift the heel of the right foot, simultaneously lifting the left toes.

4 Breathe out as you roll through the feet to bring the heels of the left foot up, while lifting the toes of the right foot.

5 Repeat this action 5 times, breathing before lowering both feet and then bringing the spine back down in one piece.

Repeat up to 5 times.

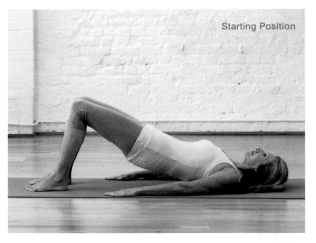
Starting Position

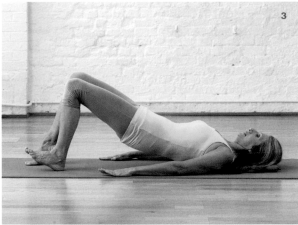

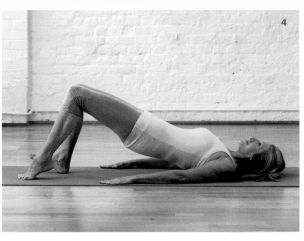

■ While your feet march, ensure that your pelvis remains still and stable. If necessary, place your hands on it to check.

■ Keep both sides of your waist long.

■ Do not lose the height of the Bridge as you march.

■ Direct your ankles forwards to prevent your feet rolling in or out.

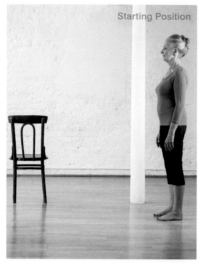
Starting Position

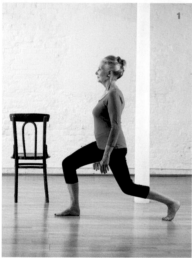
1

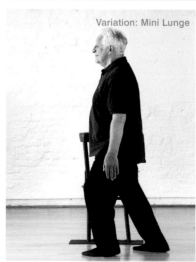
Variation: Mini Lunge

Lunge

If you break the Lunge down into component parts (stepping forwards, hip flexion/extension, knee flexion/extension), you'll see that it requires several movement skills all very appropriate to everyday life.

✱ Caution: Take advice if you have a knee, hip or ankle injury. Not suitable for hip or knee replacements. ✱

Starting Position

Stand tall, feet hip-width apart and parallel. Double check that your pelvis and spine are in neutral. Have a sturdy chair beside you if necessary.

Use an appropriate level of core connection to control your alignment and movements.

Action

1 Breathe in as you step forward with your right foot, bending the right knee and hip to about 90-degree angles, while simultaneously extending the left hip and bending the left knee parallel to the floor. As your right hip flexes your torso will naturally lean forwards slightly.

2 Breathe out as you straighten the right leg and step back to return to the Starting Position.

Repeat up to six times with each leg.

Variations: Mini (Partial) Lunge

If you find the Lunge difficult, just do a small one instead, as in the bottom left picture.

Travelling Lunge

Follow Action 1 above, but rather than returning to the Starting Position, simply step ahead with the opposite foot. Alternate legs.

✱ ■ While doing the lunges, stay lengthened and stable in the spine, keeping it in a neutral position.

■ Ensure that the knee of the leg going forwards does not go beyond the toes and stays centred over the foot; also, that the knee does not roll inwards or outwards.

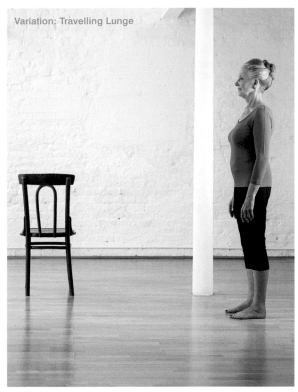
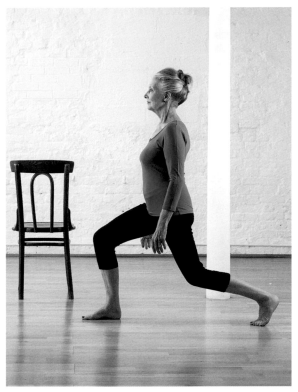
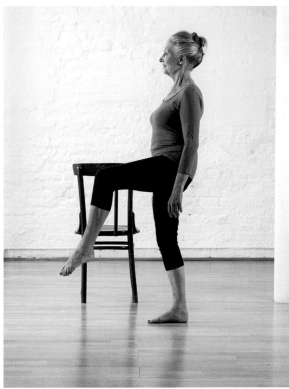
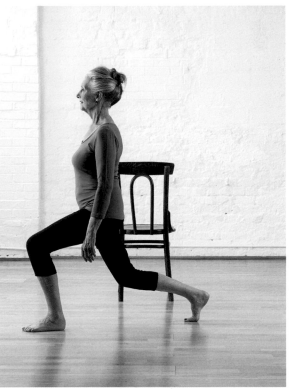

Variation: Lunge with Pick Up

A very functional version for everyday tasks! It helps to place two different objects on the floor in front of you to give yourself something to aim for. Practise the exercise first just pretending to pick up the objects, then progress to actually picking them up – this challenges your ability to balance and grasp or pinch. Note: the smaller the object, the more challenging it will be! If you use a pin, for example, you will also challenge your vision, while the pick-up action will help to improve your arm and shoulder blade movement.

Follow Action 1 on p. 96, but simultaneously hinge forward from your hips and reach with your left hand to pick up the object. Then:

2 Breathe out as you straighten the right leg and step back to return to the Starting Position.

Repeat up to 6 times on each side.

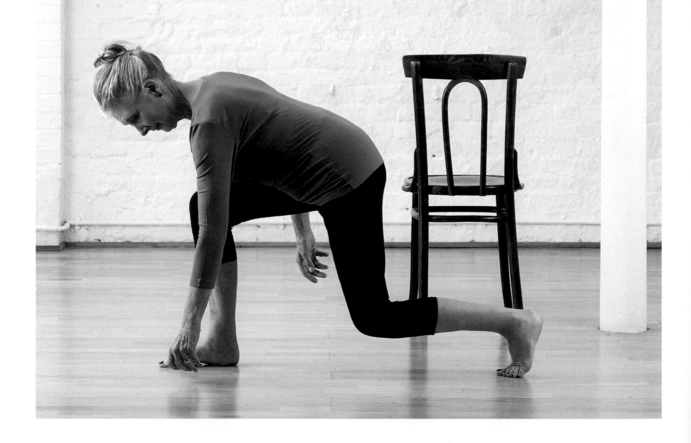

Directional Lunge

In this version you lunge in different directions – in a circle. Imagine a clock face around you and aim to touch each hour as you lunge forwards. This enhances proprioception (awareness of your joint position), vision and co-ordination.

Action

Follow the Lunge Actions 1 and 2 on p. 96, to bring you back to the Starting Position. Then:

3 Turn towards the right, say 1 o'clock, moving the right foot and then the left foot, keeping them positioned hip-width apart. When in position, perform the Lunge. Come back to the Starting Position and repeat, facing 2 o'clock, then 3 o'clock, and so on.

Advanced Variation: you may keep your left foot in the centre of the clock while you lunge, pointing your foot and turning your pelvis and trunk towards the right. Keep the left leg stationary. Stop turning once you are not able to turn your body and your foot in alignment. Repeat, turning towards the left, keeping the right leg stationary.

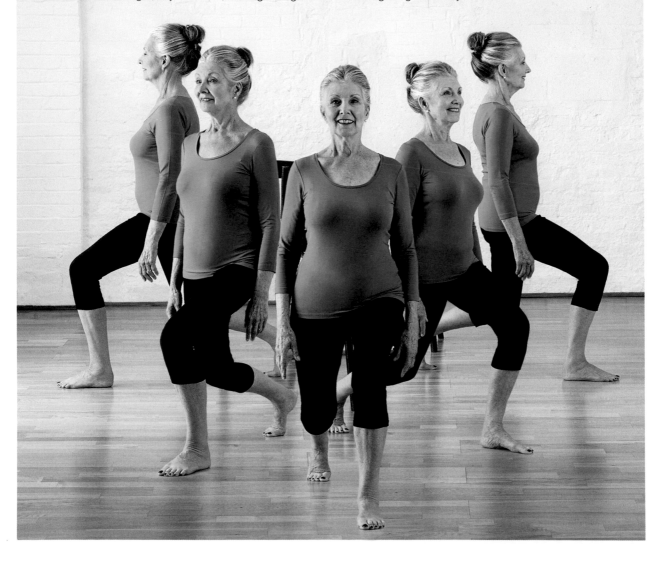

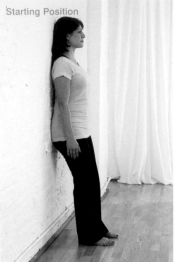

Starting Position

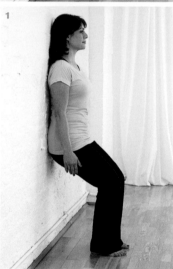

1

■ Keep whichever parts of your back that were touching the wall in the Starting Position against the wall as you slide up and down.

■ Direct your knees forwards, keeping them in line with your hips and ankles. Do not allow them to roll in or out. If necessary, place a small cushion between the knees to help you keep them hip-width apart.

■ Do not slide down too far; your pelvis should not be lower than your knees.

Sliding Down the Wall

This is such a useful exercise – it not only mobilises your hips, ankles and knees, but also strengthens your thigh muscles and teaches you good alignment.

✳ Caution: take advice if you have hip, ankle or knee problems. ✳

Starting Position

Stand tall with your back against a wall. Place your feet parallel and hip-width apart, approximately 30–60cm from the wall (when your knees are bent to a right angle, they shouldn't go beyond your toes). Take a moment to notice which parts of your back are touching the wall. (Note: it is unlikely that your head will be in contact with the wall; do not tip it back.) Feel the natural curves of your spine.

Use an appropriate level of core connection to control your alignment and movements.

Action

1 Breathe in as you bend your knees to slide your body down the wall until your thighs are almost but not parallel with the floor.

2 Breathe out as you straighten your legs and slide your body back up the wall to the Starting Position.

Repeat up to 10 times.

Variation: Wall Slides with Ribcage Closure

Here we add the challenge of a Ribcage Closure (p. 47). Your goal is to keep your ribs connected and upper back on the wall as your arms float up in front of you. It helps to hold a wooden pole or scarf. Note that the breathing pattern has changed to help you keep the ribs connected.

✳ Caution: as above, but also take advice if you have shoulder problems. ✳

Starting Position

As above, but hold the pole or scarf in front of you with both hands just wider than shoulder-width apart.

Use an appropriate level of core connection to control your alignment and movements.

Action

1 Breathe in to prepare to move.

2 Breathe out as you bend your knees to slide your body down the wall until your thighs are almost parallel with the floor. Simultaneously raise the pole or scarf up in front of you and above your head as if doing a Ribcage Closure.

3 Breathe in and maintain the position.

4 Breathe out as you straighten your legs and slide your body back up the wall to the Starting Position, simultaneously bringing your arms back down.

Repeat up to 8 times.

Variation: Wall Slides with Heel Lifts
This version challenges your ability to keep good alignment through the legs.

Action
Follow Action point 1 for Sliding down the Wall, then in this wall-squat position:

2 Breathe normally as you lift the heel of one foot, replace it, then repeat with the other foot.

3 Repeat 3 times, then:

4 Breathe out as you straighten your legs and slide your body back up the wall to the Starting Position.

Repeat the sequence 3 times.

In addition to the points opposite, for the Variation with Rib Cage Closure:

■ Depending on your level of flexibility, your arms will probably not reach the wall in step 2. Do not force them back.

■ As your arms float up in front of you, do not allow your upper back to arch away from the wall.

For the Variation with Heel Lifts:

■ Send your ankle directly forwards as your heel lifts to prevent your foot rolling in or out.

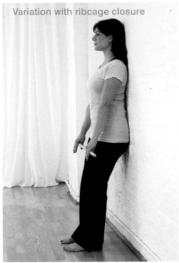

Variation with ribcage closure

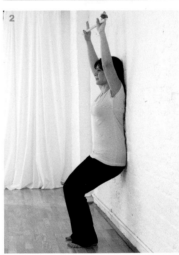

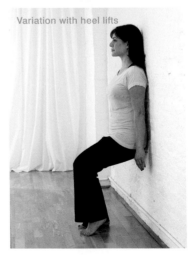

Variation with heel lifts

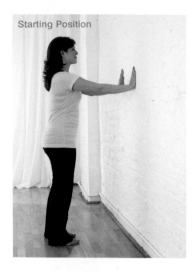

Starting Position

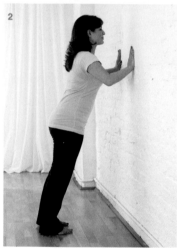

2

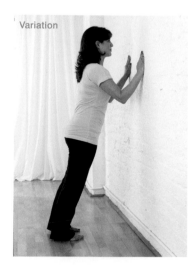

Variation

Wall Push-ups

A gentle, but effective, exercise for strengthening the arms. The two versions here target both the triceps and biceps.

✳ Caution: take medical advice if you have fractured your wrist within the last 2–3 months; you should not feel any pain with the movement. ✳

Starting Position

Stand tall, facing a wall as far away as you need to be so that only your fingertips touch the wall. Have your arms just less than shoulder-width apart and your feet either hip-width apart or in Pilates Stance (p. 35).

Use an appropriate level of core connection to control your alignment and movements.

Action

1 Breathe in to prepare, and lengthen up through the spine.

2 Breathe out as you bend your elbows outwards, rolling sequentially through your wrists and hands to lean your body forwards towards the wall. Move your trunk as one piece, keeping your body straight (as if you have swallowed a stick).

3 Breathe in to hold the position.

4 Breathe out as you press back out to the Starting Position.

Repeat 8 times.

Variation

As above, but bend your elbows directly downwards.

* ■ Keep your body long and strong; do not collapse in the middle, keep the ribs connected.

■ Bend your elbows downwards, but remember to stay open across your collarbones.

■ Keep your head and neck in line with the rest of your body.

■ You will have to hinge from your ankle joint to achieve the right movement.

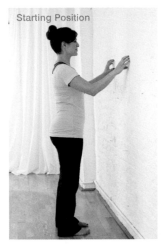
Starting Position

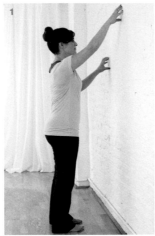
1

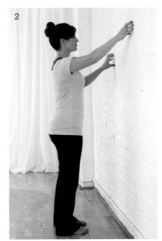
2

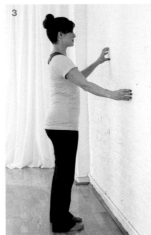
3

Walking on the Wall Up and Down

The aim of this exercise is to mobilise your shoulders. It is not as impossible as the name suggests!

Starting Position

Stand tall at a comfortable distance from the wall with your feet hip-width apart, arms bent at the elbows (which are facing downwards) and fingertips just touching the wall.

Use an appropriate level of core connection to control your alignment and movements.

Action

Breathe normally throughout.

1 Move the fingers of one hand in a walking action along the wall, travelling upwards.

2 Walk the fingers back down to the starting position. Repeat up to 5 times with each arm.

3 Now walk your fingers to take one arm to the side.

4 Walk your fingers back to the starting position and repeat the sequence with the other arm.

Variations

■ Walk your fingers out to the side then in an arc up the wall before returning to the Starting Position.

■ Walk one hand upwards and the other downwards at the same time.

Once you become good at this exercise, you can move your feet closer to the wall.

■ Maintain the correct standing position and the distance between the shoulders and the ears.

■ Sense the movement of the shoulder blades without any squeezing or rounding.

■ Take care not to overreach.

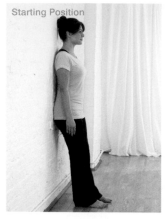
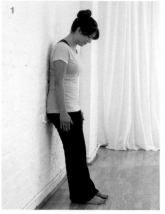
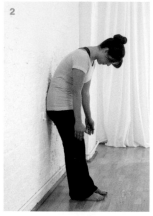
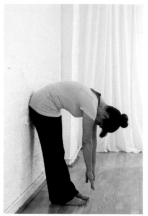

Starting Position   1   2

Roll-downs Against the Wall

Using a wall enables you to feel the wheeling, segmental movement of the spine both on the way down and on the way back up. Fabulous for mobilising the spine and hips.

✳ Caution: avoid if you have been diagnosed with osteoporosis. Take advice if you have had a hip replacement in the last 6–12 weeks or have back problems. ✳

Starting Position

Stand tall with your back against a wall. Place your feet parallel and hip-width apart, approximately 30–60cm from the wall. If you know that you're not very flexible, bend your knees very slightly. As with Sliding Down the Wall (p. 100), take a moment to feel the natural curves of the spine, noticing which parts of your back are touching the wall. Depending on your posture, your head may or may not be in contact with the wall; do not force it back.

Use an appropriate level of core connection to control your alignment and movements.

Action

1 Breathe in as you lengthen the back of your neck and nod your head forwards.

2 Breathe out as you continue to roll your entire spine forwards and down. Create length in the spine as you do so. When you have rolled as far as you can with your spine, you may bend from the hips.

3 Breathe in at the bottom of the Roll-down.

4 Breathe out as you roll your pelvis under and, bone by bone, restack the spine back up the wall to stand tall.

Repeat up to 5 times.

✳ ■ Take an extra breath on the way down/way up, if you need to.

■ Take care not to collapse forwards; use your deep abdominal muscles to support your lengthened spine.

■ It helps to have an image of a large ball that you need to go up and over.

Dumb Waiter

A very important exercise as it helps to rebalance the movement of your upper arm in relation to your shoulder blades. It also helps to release and open the front of your chest and shoulders.

Starting Position

Either: Stand tall on the floor (not on your mat). Bend your elbows to an approximate right angle, have your upper arm positioned vertically and your forearm lengthening forwards horizontally. Turn your palms to face upwards (like a waiter holding a tray).

Or: Sit upright on a sturdy, armless chair, with feet grounded hip-width apart on the floor.

Use an appropriate level of core connection to control your alignment and movements.

Action

1 Breathe in as you turn your arms outwards from the shoulder joint, reaching your forearms wide. Keep your elbows directly underneath your shoulders.

2 Breathe out as you return the arms back to the Starting Position.

Repeat up to 6 times.

Variation: Using Weights

You may use light hand weights up to 1–3kg per weight (depending on your ability). If you are using weights, the actions remain the same, but it is best to work one arm at time. If you are using a hand-held weight, hold it with your palm facing inwards; if your weight wraps around your wrist, palms may face upwards, as above.

Variation: Adding Medial Rotation

In this version, you will add the extra movement of turning in the arm at the shoulder. You will need to remember everything you learned in Thumb Rolls (p. 77). Once again, work one arm at a time. To ensure you are moving the arm correctly and to deter any rounding of the shoulders, place the other hand on top of your shoulder.

Starting Position

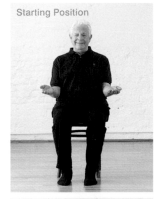

1

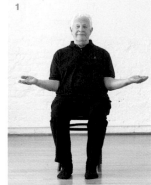

Variation using weights

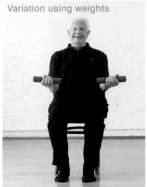

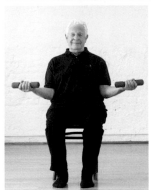

Variation with medial rotation

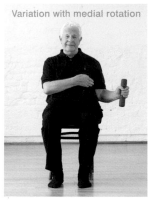

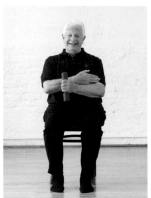

* ■ Move your arm from the shoulder joint.

■ Do not squeeze your shoulder blades together.

■ Stay open across your collarbones and across your upper back.

■ Keep your fingers and hands lengthened, wrists long and strong.

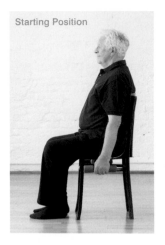
Starting Position

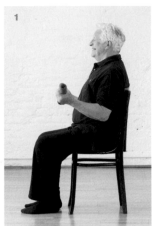
1

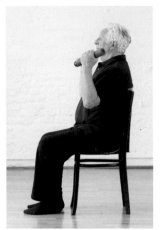

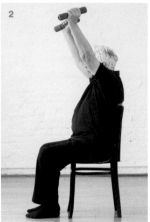
2

Biceps Press

It is good to add free weights to the programme as they can help build more tone in your muscles, as well as strength in your bones. The rule of thumb is that you should practise an exercise first without weights (or perhaps with a tennis ball) to master your technique, then with a light weight, progressing to heavier weights as long as your technique remains good. In Biceps Press you are also mobilising your elbow and shoulder joints.

✳ Caution: take advice if you have wrist, elbow or shoulder problems. Avoid taking your arms above your head when standing if you have heart or blood pressure problems. ✳

Starting Position

Sit on a sturdy, armless chair or stand tall holding a light weight or tennis ball in each hand, arms lengthened down by your sides, palms facing your body.

Use an appropriate level of core connection to control your alignment and movements.

Action

1 Breathe in as you bend your elbows and turn your palms up, drawing your hands up towards your shoulders. The palms end up facing the body.

2 Breathe out as you straighten your elbows and raise the arms upwards overhead. As you do so, the palms will turn towards one another.

3 Breathe in as you lower your arms, drawing your hands back down towards your shoulder joints, palms back facing the body.

4 Breathe out as you straighten and lower the arms, returning them to the Starting Position.

Repeat 8 times.

✳ ■ As the arms reach overhead, take care to maintain your neutral alignment.

■ Do not allow the ribs to flare or the back to arch.

■ Ensure correct alignment at the wrist and elbow joints.

■ When straightening the arms, avoid locking the elbows.

Triceps

This useful exercise uses hand-held weights which help tone the upper arms and mobilise your elbow joints. The added weight also improves bone density.

✳ Caution: take advice if you have hand, wrist, elbow or shoulder problems. ✳

Starting Position
The Relaxation Position. Hold a tennis ball or weight (up to 2kg) in your right hand with that arm straight above your right shoulder joint, palm facing forwards. Your left arm is bent, and supports the right arm just behind the elbow.

Use an appropriate level of core connection to control your alignment and movements.

Action
1 Breathe in as you bend your right elbow, directing the hand towards the left elbow.

2 Breathe out as you straighten the elbow, returning the arm to the Starting Position.

Repeat up to 10 times, then repeat with the other arm.

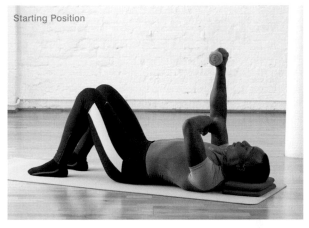

Starting Position

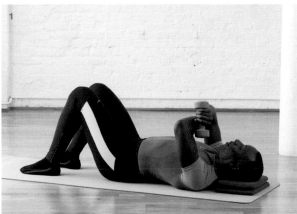

✳ ■ Your upper arm must remain still throughout. Ensure that the movement comes from your elbow and not your shoulder joint.

■ Stay in control of the movements.

■ Keep your wrists long and strong and in good alignment.

■ Take care not to overextend the arm as you straighten it.

■ If your arm starts to shake or you feel you are losing your technique or control, STOP. You can always return to the exercise later to complete the repetitions.

Dart

This is a 'must-do' exercise which mobilises the spine in extension and strengthens your upper-back muscles, vital for maintaining good posture. There is a lot happening at once here, so read through several times before trying it.

✱ Caution: take advice if you have back problems or if you have been diagnosed with spinal stenosis – you may wish to place a small cushion under your waist. ✱

Starting Position

Lie prone with a cushion underneath the forehead if you wish. Lengthen your arms down by your sides, resting on the mat, palms facing upwards; your legs are also lengthened, the base of the big toes touching. If you have osteoporosis, you may place a flat cushion under your abdomen.

Use an appropriate level of core connection to control your alignment and movements.

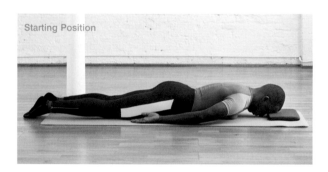

Starting Position

Action

1 Breathe in to prepare to move.

2 Breathe out as you start to extend the upper spine, lengthening and lifting first your head, then neck, then upper spine one vertebra at a time. Simultaneously draw your legs together, connecting the inner thighs to bring them into a parallel position. At the same time, lengthen the arms away and lift them slightly as they turn outwards so that the palms now face your body.

3 Breathe in and maintain this lengthened position.

4 Breathe out as you sequentially return the upper back, then neck, then head to the mat, while simultaneously relaxing your legs and turning your arms back to the Starting Position.

Repeat up to 10 times.

Variation: the Dart may also be done with the legs slightly wider than hip-width apart and turned out from the hips.

■ Take care not to tip your head back too far, keeping your gaze down throughout.

■ Ensure the right order of events: first the head lifts, then the neck and, when they are in line with the upper spine, the upper spine extends. Your ribs stay connected down into your waist.

■ Do not be tempted to lift the legs – they stay grounded.

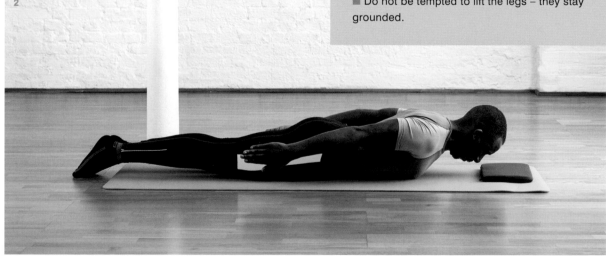

2

Full Star

This will mobilise your spine, shoulder and hip joints. You should be confident with Star Preparation and Cobra Preparation with Arm Slide (pp. 49 and 61) before attempting it.

✱ Caution: take advice if you have back or shoulder problems. Avoid if you have been diagnosed with stenosis of the spine. ✱

Starting Position

Lie prone on your mat, your pelvis and lumbar spine in neutral. Have your legs slightly wider than hip-width apart and turned out from the hips, arms reaching above you, resting on the mat, slightly wider than shoulder-width apart and palms down. If you have osteoporosis, you may place a flat cushion under your abdomen to help you maintain neutral.

Use an appropriate level of core connection to control your alignment and movements.

Action

1 Breathe in to prepare to move.

2 Breathe out as you sequentially lift your head, neck and upper spine into a Diamond/Dart position (see opposite). Keep your ribs down and shine your breastbone forwards.

3 Breathe in and lengthen through the spine.

4 Breathe out as you lengthen and lift opposite arm and leg slightly off the mat without disturbing your spine or pelvis.

5 Breathe in as you lower your arm and leg back down to the mat, but keep your upper-back extension.

Repeat up to 10 times, alternating arms and legs, then lengthen back down to the Starting Position.

Variation: you may turn the palms to face each other, if this is more comfortable for your shoulders.

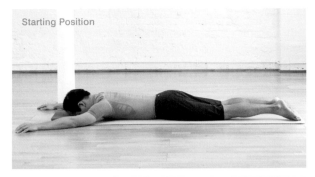
Starting Position

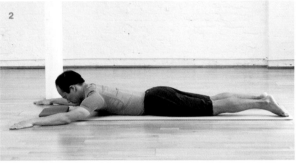
2

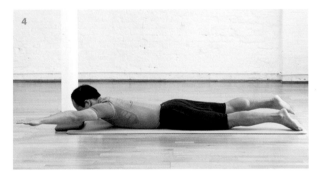
4

✱ ■ Do not overreach with your arms; keep the width across your shoulders and the distance between your ears and shoulders.

■ Lift your arm and leg only as high as you can while maintaining a still and stable pelvis and spine.

■ Keep the arms and legs fully lengthened, but avoid locking the elbows and knees throughout.

Lizard

Here is another back-extension exercise, but this time with an added rotational element and, in Version 2, a leg action. It involves good body awareness to get the co-ordination right.

✴ Caution: take advice if you have back problems. Avoid if you have been diagnosed with stenosis of the spine. ✴

Starting Position

Lie prone. Rest your forehead on the mat or a folded towel. Your legs should be straight, slightly wider than hip-width apart and turned out from the hips; bend your elbows and position your hands slightly wider than, and above, your shoulders, palms facing down. Make sure that your shoulders are released and your collarbones are wide. If you have osteoporosis, you may place a flat cushion under your abdomen to help you maintain neutral.

Use an appropriate level of core connection to control your alignment and movements.

Action

1 Breathe in to prepare.

2 Breathe out as you open your left shoulder by pressing gently on your left hand, lifting and rotating your head, spine and ribs to the left until you are looking over your left shoulder.

3 Breathe into that open side and hold the position.

4 Breathe out and slowly return to the Starting Position, moving first through your ribs and shoulders and, finally, bringing your head back to rest.

Repeat, rotating to the right side. Repeat up to 8 times.

Lizard – Variation

We can now add the leg action to mobilise your knee and gently lengthen the front of your thighs.

Follow Action points 1 and 2 above, then:

3 Breathe in as you bend your right knee, directing your foot towards your left shoulder. The knee stays on the mat. Proceed to Action point 4 above.

Repeat with the other side and leg. Repeat up to 4 times.

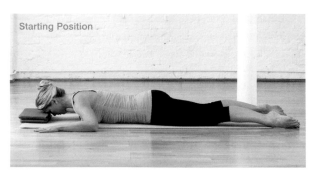
Starting Position

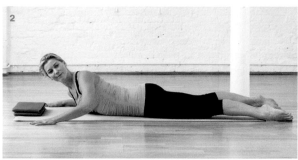
2

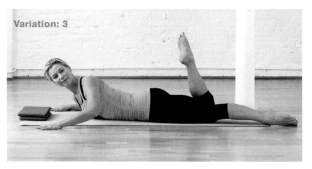
Variation: 3

■ Keep your pelvis grounded and centred throughout.

■ Press gently through your arm to help your upper body rotation, but avoid pushing hard.

■ Do not overextend your neck by turning your head further than feels comfortable.

■ Keep collarbones wide and open.

■ Control your return; do not collapse back down.

■ With Version 2, return the leg to the Starting Position precisely each time.

Full Table-top

This challenges your ability to move your limbs independently, while staying stable. You must remain in control to do it well, so follow the directions carefully. It makes sense to practise Table-top Preparation (p. 50) before attempting this.

✳ Caution: take advice if you have shoulder problems or have recently had breast cancer surgery. ✳

Starting Position
Four-point Kneeling Position.

Use an appropriate level of core connection to control your alignment and movements.

Action
1 Breathe in to prepare to move.

2 Breathe out as you slide one leg behind you, directly in line with your hip, simultaneously lengthening and sliding the opposite hand away along the mat in line with your shoulder. Your softly pointed foot will remain in contact with the mat, your pelvis and spine still and stable.

3 Breathe in as you lengthen and lift your leg to hip height. Simultaneously raise the opposite arm forwards, ideally to shoulder height. Once again, stay lengthened and stable in your trunk.

4 Breathe out as you lower your hand and foot to the mat.

5 Breathe in as you return your arm and leg back to the Starting Position, still keeping your spine and pelvis still.

Repeat up to 5 times on each side, alternating opposite arms and legs.

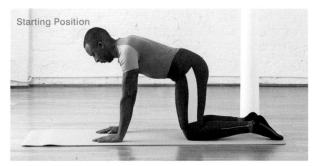

Starting Position

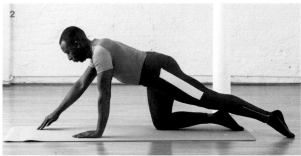

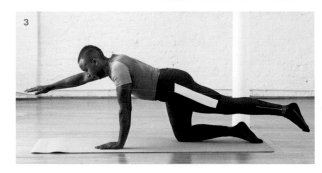

✳ Your arm should ideally rise to the height of your shoulder, your leg to the height of your hip, but do not disturb the pelvis or spine.

■ Maintain a distance between your ears and shoulders, collarbones remaining wide and open.

■ Keep both sides of your waist equally lengthened.

■ Your pelvis should stay square to the mat; do not allow it to twist or dip.

■ Keep your neck lengthened and your head in line with your spine; do not allow it to drop.

Climb A Tree Preparation

A gentle way to mobilise the hip and knee and lengthen the back of the thigh.

✱ Caution: take advice if you have knee or hip problems. ✱

Starting Position

The Relaxation Position. Single-knee-fold your left leg (p. 44). Draw the leg in as far as possible without disturbing the neutral alignment of the pelvis. Softly point your foot. Lightly clasp your hands behind your left thigh. If you cannot reach easily, use a towel, scarf or stretch band.

Use an appropriate level of core connection to control your alignment and movements.

Action

1 Breathe in to prepare to move.

2 Breathe out as you straighten your left leg, keeping your pelvis in neutral.

3 Breathe in as you bend the knee again to return to the Starting Position. Repeat up to 5 times and then repeat on the other leg.

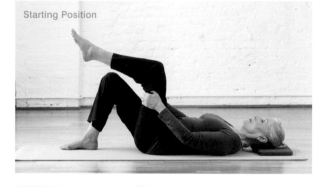

Starting Position

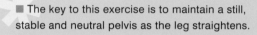

■ The key to this exercise is to maintain a still, stable and neutral pelvis as the leg straightens.

■ Try to keep the upper part of the bending/straightening leg still.

■ Fully straighten the leg, but avoid locking out the knee.

■ Keep the foot, ankle, knee and hip in alignment.

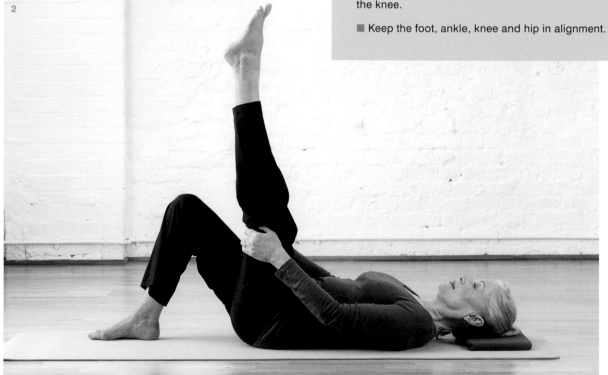

2

Pray

This exercise will improve your shoulder and wrist mobility and strength.

✳ Caution: take advice if you have wrist or shoulder problems. ✳

Starting Position

Sit tall on a sturdy chair (or stand tall). Have your feet hip-width apart, arms bent at the elbows and hands together in a prayer position, thumbs facing the centre of your chest (about a hand's distance away from the chest).

Use an appropriate level of core connection to control your alignment and movements.

Action

1 Breathe in as you move both arms overhead, keeping your hands together in the prayer shape.

2 Breathe out as you lower your arms to the Starting Position, then as low as you can while keeping the heels of your hands together.

3 Breathe in and return to the Starting Position.

Repeat up to 10 times.

■ Maintain good posture throughout, staying lengthened on both sides of your waist.

■ Maintain the distance between ears and shoulders.

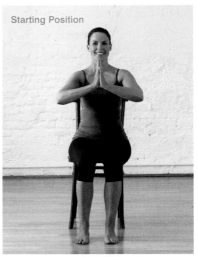

Starting Position

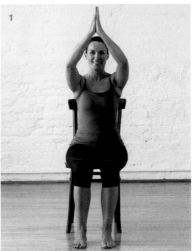

1

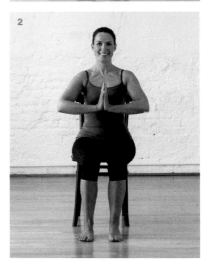

2

Arm Swing

This exercise not only mobilises your shoulders, but will also help with your walking pattern.

✻ Caution: take advice if you have shoulder problems. ✻

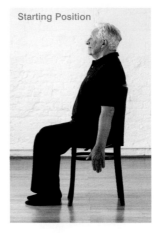
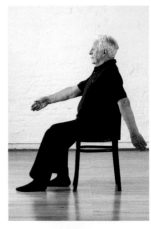

Starting Position

Starting Position
Either sit tall on an armless chair or stand tall, feet hip-width apart and arms down by your sides.

Use an appropriate level of core connection to control your alignment and movements.

Action
Breathe normally throughout.

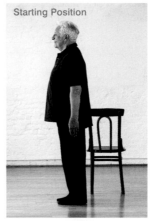
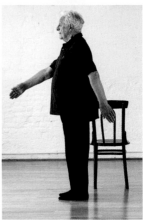

Starting Position

Move one arm forwards and the other backwards. Let the thumb lead the forwards arm movement, while the little finger leads the backwards arm movement. Sense a pendulum movement, drawing a semi arc with the fingers. Keep your body stable and aligned, looking straight ahead.

Repeat 12 times.

Variation: Arm Swing in an Offset Stance Position
As the movement improves, place one foot forwards in an offset stance position.

Follow the directions above, then swap to place the other foot forwards.

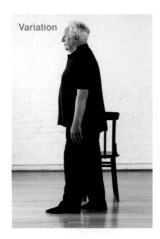
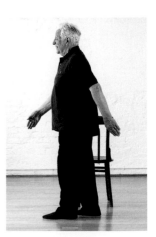

Variation

Variation: in the above offset stance position, follow all the directions above, but as you move your arms, rotate your head and trunk, turning in the same direction as the backwards moving arm.

✱ ■ Remember to lengthen up at all times, but allow your arms to swing freely.

■ If you are turning, remember what you learned in Waist Twists (p. 64).

Side-lying Legs – Lift and Lower

This exercise mobilises your hip joints, but if you use ankle weights, (up to 1kg for each weight) you will strengthen your gluteals and outer-thigh muscles. Practise first without weights. Getting the Starting Position right is vital.

✱ Caution: take advice if you have hip, back or knee problems. ✱

Starting Position

Side-lying on your left side, extend your left arm in line with the spine so that you can rest your head on it. Place a flat pillow or folded towel there to keep the head and spine in alignment. Place your right hand on the mat on front of your ribcage, elbow bent (this arm will help support you). Bend both legs in front of you, so that the hips and knees are at approximately 90 degrees. With control, lengthen and lift your right leg. Straighten the knee and bring the leg, in parallel, in line with your spine at hip height. Flex your foot, lengthening through the heel.

Use an appropriate level of core connection to control your alignment and movements.

Action

1 Breathe in to prepare to move.

2 Breathe out as you lift your right leg directly upwards. Lift the leg up as far as you can without disturbing the pelvis and spine.

3 Breathe in as you lower the leg back to hip height with control. Do not lower the working leg below hip height.

Repeat 10 times before bending the right leg and bringing it safely back to rest on the left. Always finish by bending the knee and placing it back onto the 'resting' leg.

Repeat on the other side.

Variation: this exercise (and those on pp. 116-117) may be done with the leg slightly turned in from the hip. If you do this, ensure that the internal rotation takes place from the hip joint and not the knee or ankle joint. (Avoid this version if you have had a hip replacement.)

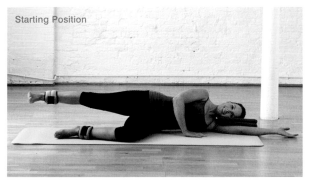
Starting Position

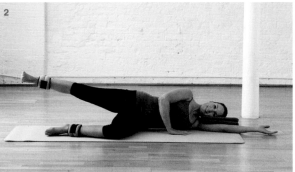
2

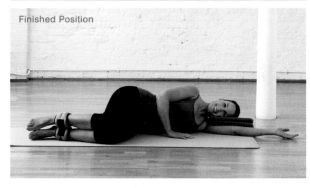
Finished Position

■ For most people, the leg will only lift a few centimetres before the pelvis and spine move, so take care not to lift too high.

■ Keep both sides of your waist lifted and lengthened.

■ Avoid placing too much weight on your top arm.

■ Do not roll forwards or back. Your chest stays open.

■ Really lengthen the heel away from the hip as you lift.

Side-lying Knee Cross-overs

This mobilises the hip joint while strengthening the supporting muscles. It's the sister/brother exercise to Oyster (p. 51).

✱ Caution: take advice if you are recovering from a hip-replacement operation. ✱

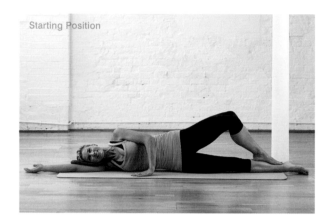

Starting Position

Starting Position

Side-lying on your right side with your head resting on your outstretched right arm, palm facing up; use a flat cushion or folded towel to bring your head in line with the neck and spine, if needed. Your right leg should be straight in line with your body, your left knee bent, the left foot resting on the right knee or calf. Double-check that your pelvis and spine are in neutral. Your left hand should be in front of your chest to support you and help your balance.

Use an appropriate level of core connection to control your alignment and movements.

Action

1 Breathe in to prepare to move.

2 Breathe out as you cross the left knee over the right leg and down towards the floor.

3 Breathe in as you lift the left knee, keeping the left foot on the right knee or calf, and return it to the Starting Position. Repeat 10 times, then turn over and repeat on the other side.

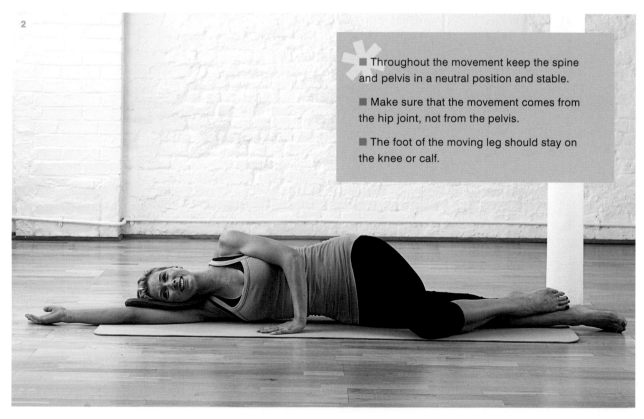

2

✱ ■ Throughout the movement keep the spine and pelvis in a neutral position and stable.

■ Make sure that the movement comes from the hip joint, not from the pelvis.

■ The foot of the moving leg should stay on the knee or calf.

Side-lying Bicycle

This will mobilise your hip and knee and challenge your core stability. You will probably find the reverse cycle a little difficult to begin with, which is great for your co-ordination skills!

✻ Caution: take advice if you have back, hip or knee problems. ✻

Starting Position

Side-lying on your left side, left arm outstretched in line with your spine. Hinge both legs forwards a little from the hips. Bend your right arm at the elbow and place the hand in front of your chest. Rest your head on your extended arm (use a flat cushion/folded towel to keep it in line with your spine) and extend your legs in line with your spine. With control, lengthen and lift your right leg to hip height.

Use an appropriate level of core connection to control your alignment and movements.

Action

1 Breathe in as you lengthen your right leg slightly behind you, still at hip height and taking care not to disturb the pelvis or spine.

2 Breathe out as you bend your right knee, your heel reaching towards the back of the thigh; then, moving from the hip, carry the leg forwards, keeping the knee bent.

3 Breathe in as you straighten your right knee (it is still at hip height and your pelvis and spine are still stable).

4 Breathe out as you return the right leg back behind your pelvis.

Repeat 3 times and reverse the movement.

5 Breathe in as your right leg reaches forwards at hip height.

6 Breathe out as you bend the knee and then, moving from the hip joint, carry the leg backwards.

7 Breathe in as you straighten the knee, then bring the leg forwards in line with your hip.

Repeat 3 times. Then turn over to repeat on the other side.

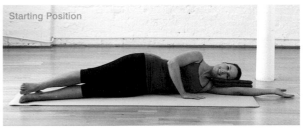

Starting Position

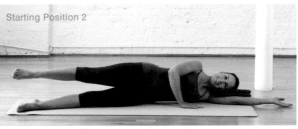

Starting Position 2

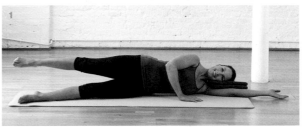

1

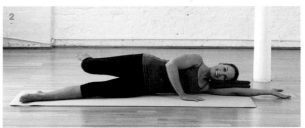

2

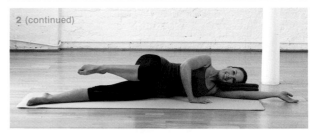

2 (continued)

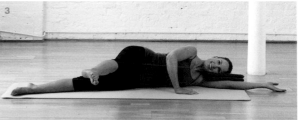

3

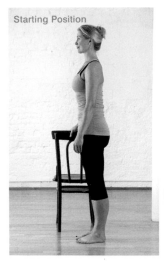 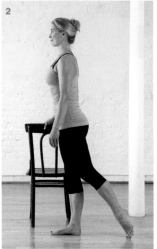 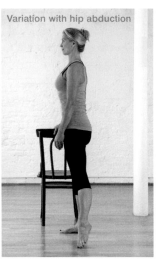 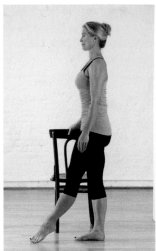

Starting Position   2   Variation with hip abduction

Standing Star

These exercises challenge your balance while mobilising the spine and opening the hip joint. You'll need to multitask here and remember what you learned in Star Preparation and Side Reach (pp. 49 and 71).

To help, we have broken the exercise down, so that you can layer on the next movement when you feel ready.

✳ Caution: Take advice if you have balance problems. ✳

Starting Position

Stand tall on the floor (not the mat), feet hip-width apart and parallel. Stand by a chair if you are not sure of your balance.

Use an appropriate level of core connection to control your alignment and movements.

Action

1 Breathe in to prepare, lengthen up through the spine and transfer your weight onto your right foot with minimal disturbance to the pelvis and spine.

2 Breathe out as you lengthen your left foot away behind you, just a little, keeping your pelvis square to the front. Your foot stays in contact with the floor although your heel lifts. Keep the leg in parallel if you can.

3 Breathe in and bring the foot back in line.

4 Repeat 5 times with each leg.

Variation – adding weights: the above exercise may be done wearing light ankle weights. This makes it especially good for osteoporosis and hip health.

Variation – adding hip abduction and flexion: here you take the leg out to the side, and then in front.

✳ ■ Keep both sides of your waist equally long as the leg moves.

■ Try not to tip forwards as the leg moves.

■ Alternate the leg you start with each time you do the exercise.

Standing Star plus Side Reach

Moving on from Standing Star, we're adding lateral flexion of the spine with a Side Reach. This is challenging, as you must control both the movement of the spine and the position of the pelvis and all on a reduced base of support.

✱ Caution: take advice if you have problems with your balance. ✱

Starting Position

Follow the Starting Position and Actions opposite, so that you are standing on your right foot and your left foot is lengthened away behind.

Use an appropriate level of core connection to control your alignment and movements.

Action

1 Breathe in to prepare to move, and float your left arm up, keeping it in front of you.

2 Breathe out as you sequentially reach your head, neck and upper spine to the right.

3 Breathe into the ribs on the open side and hold the position.

4 Breathe out as you lengthen and reach back up to the centre, and lower the arm with control.

5 Repeat the Side Reach now to the left.

6 Repeat the sequence with the left leg behind you.

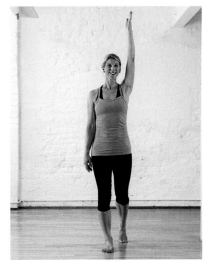

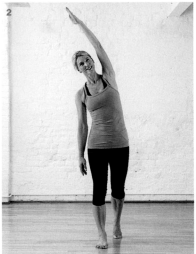

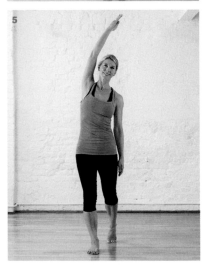

✱
■ When you float your arm up it should stay slightly in front of you, the palm turning to face forwards as you lift.

■ When you reach over to the side, lift and lengthen both sides of your waist.

■ Try to reach directly to the side and not shift forwards or back.

STANDING SIDE STRETCHES

We have given you two great exercises here that will open out the sides of your body and your hip joints.

Standing Side Stretch on a Step

✱ Caution: take advice if you have hip or balance problems. ✱

Starting Position
Stand tall in front of a step or low box. With control, knee-fold your right leg up and place your foot on the step. As you step up, lunge forwards slightly, so the heel of your left foot lifts.

Use an appropriate level of core connection to control your alignment and movements.

Action
1 Breathe in to prepare to move and float your left arm up slightly in front of you.

2 Breathe out as you reach first your head, then neck, then spine up and over to the right (as for Side Reach, p. 70).

3 Breathe in there.

4 Breathe out as you reach up and back to the centre.

5 Breathe in and lower your arm.

6 Repeat the stretch on the other side.

Repeat twice, stretching to each side, then change legs and repeat the sequence.

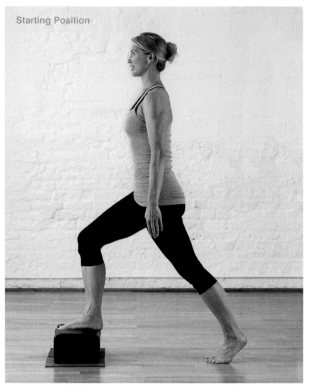

Starting Position

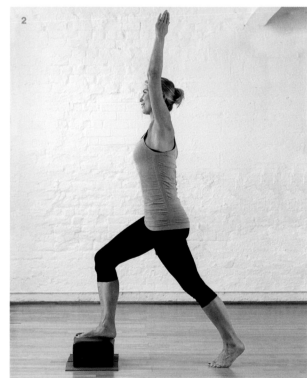

2

✱
■ Keep your pelvis centred and square at all times.

■ Remember what you learned in Floating Arms (p. 52).

Standing Side Stretch with Cross-over Leg

In this exercise you achieve a fabulous stretch down the whole side of your body and leg.

✳ Caution: take advice if you have hip or balance problems. Avoid if you have had a hip replacement in the last 6–12 weeks. ✳

Starting Position

Stand tall on the floor (not the mat). Have a sturdy chair near by, if necessary. Cross your right foot over your left.

Use an appropriate level of core connection to control your alignment and movements.

Action

1 Breathe in to prepare to move and float your right arm up.

2 Breathe out as you stretch up and over to the left, taking care not to shift your pelvis to the right as you do so.

3 Breathe in and hold the stretch.

4 Breathe out as you reach up and back to the centre.

5 Breathe in as you lower your arm.

6 Repeat the stretch on the other side.

Repeat the sequence twice before repeating with the left foot crossed over the right.

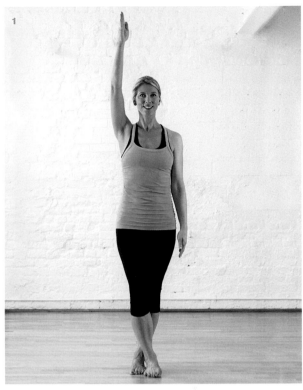

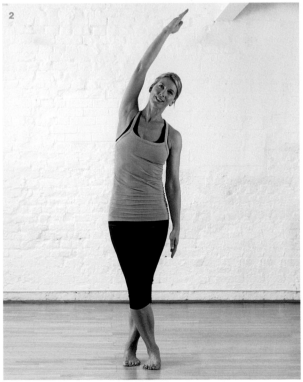

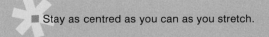

■ Stay as centred as you can as you stretch.

Crawling

An unusual exercise, but very effective at improving shoulder, hip and spine function. It will challenge your co-ordination, as well as your ability to control the alignment and movement of the pelvis and spine in simple everyday movements such as walking. You will need some clear floor space with a cushioned surface. (Beware of carpet burn – wear something that covers your knees!) This is a free-flowing natural movement sequence, but do not forget your Pilates principles.

✴ Caution: avoid if you have knee problems or have recently had a breast operation. ✴

Starting Position
Four-point Kneeling Position.

Use an appropriate level of core connection to control your alignment and movements.

Action
Breathe normally throughout.

1 Move the right hand forwards and, simultaneously, move the left knee forwards in a crawling action.

2 Move the left hand and the right knee together. Travel across the room until you reach the wall or an obstacle.

3 Crawl backwards to where you started.

Repeat 3 times (depending on the size of your room!).

Variation: crawl in a diagonal line to reach the right corner of the room. Crawl backwards on the same diagonal. Repeat, moving towards the left corner of the room.

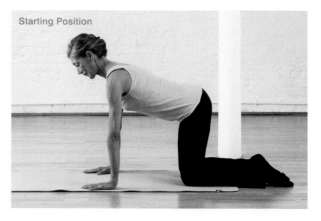

Starting Position

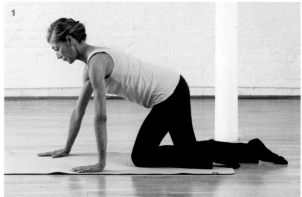

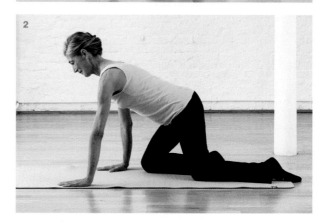

STANDING-BALANCE EXERCISES

In this series of exercises we will be gradually reducing your base of support, thus challenging your balance skills. Remember that standing tall should be an active, not static, exercise. Spend about 20–30 seconds or so (no need to look at the clock) in each position before trying the next. It makes sense to clear the area and stand by a wall or sturdy chair when you practise these exercises. Ideally, they should be done barefoot, you can wear lightweight and supportive shoes with flexible, non-slip soles.

✳ Caution: take advice if you have vestibular or eye problems. ✳

Starting Position
Stand tall with your feet together. Have a chair alongside you if you wish.

Use an appropriate level of core connection to control your alignment and movements.

Action
Breathe normally throughout.

1 Move your right foot forwards just a little (it should stay close to your left foot) and stand tall. Breathe.

2 Bring your foot back in line with the other, then bring your left foot forwards.

3 Bring your feet back to the Starting Position, then place your right foot in the same line but further forwards, so the inside of your right heel is just touching the edge of your left big toe.

4 Repeat with the left foot forwards.

5 Now for the hardest challenge: place your right foot immediately in front of your left, heel to toes.

6 Repeat with the other foot in front. Now repeat the whole series, but add an arm swing (p. 114).

✳ ■ Keep your gaze forwards and soft. Remember to blink!

■ Feel as though you are growing taller with every breath.

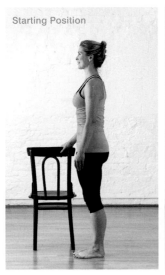
Starting Position

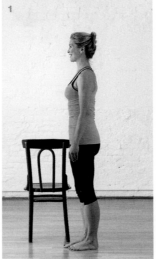
1

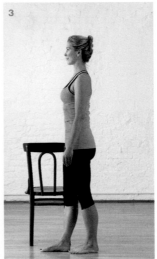
3

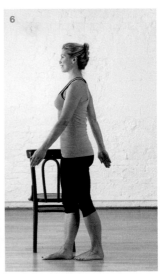
6

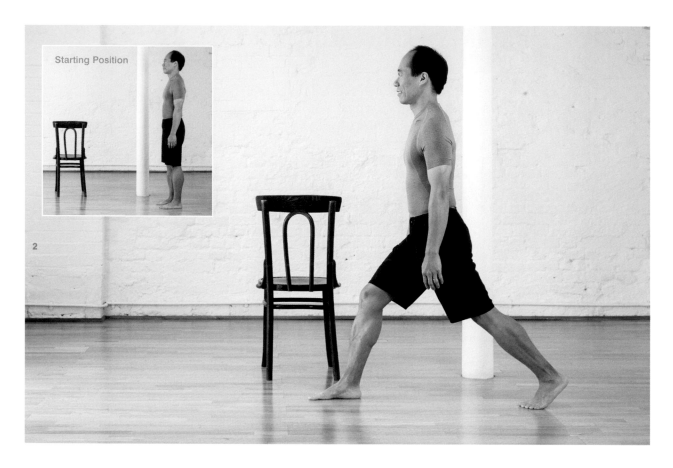

Starting Position

2

Long Stride

This will help improve your walking posture and balance, mobilising the joints of your lower limbs and strengthening their muscles. Wear light, flexible, non-slip, supportive shoes, if you wish.

Starting Position

Stand tall, feet just wider than hip-width apart and parallel. Check your alignment – you should be in neutral. Have a chair alongside if you wish.

Use an appropriate level of core connection to control your alignment and movements.

Action

You might wish to practise this a few times just breathing normally, before adding the breathing pattern.

1 Breathe in to prepare your body to move.

2 Breathe out as you move the right foot forwards in a long step/stride.

3 Breathe in as you touch the floor with your front right foot and stop in the position, then immediately step back, breathing out as you move the right foot back to the Starting Position.

Repeat 5 times, then start again, stepping forwards with the left foot.

■ While moving the foot forwards, stay lengthened in the spine and avoid shifting the weight backwards.

■ Once you have placed the foot forwards, ensure the weight is evenly distributed.

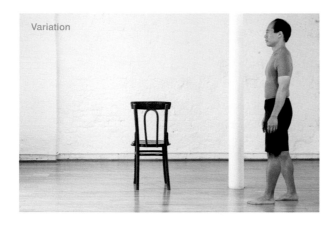

Variation

Variation: you may start with one foot forward (offset) in a Stance Position. Before you begin the Actions opposite, check that your weight is evenly distributed on both feet.

Repeat the Action points opposite, stepping forwards with the back foot, then stepping back into the Starting Position. Repeat 5 times, then change legs.

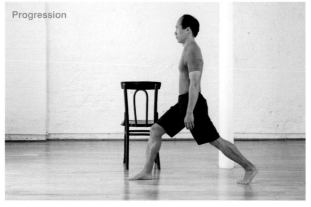

Progression

Progressions – as a progression of the foot-forwards position, you can travel forwards:

Step ahead with the back foot, with a stop to balance, before moving the foot that is now back.

More challenging: walking with Long Stride, keep stepping ahead with the back foot without stopping. Imagine that you are stamping on little dots.

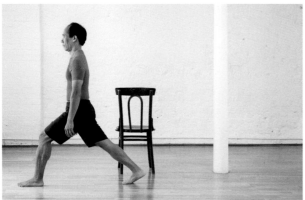

WEIGHT-TRANSFER EXERCISES

The following series of exercises will help improve your balance in different directions. Wear light, flexible, supportive non-slip shoes if you wish.

Starting Position

Stand tall behind a sturdy chair with your feet hip-width apart. Place both hands on the chair.

Use an appropriate level of core connection to control your alignment and movements.

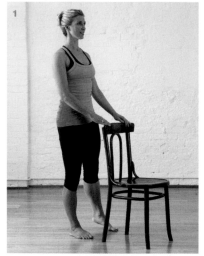

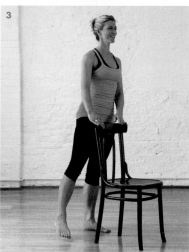

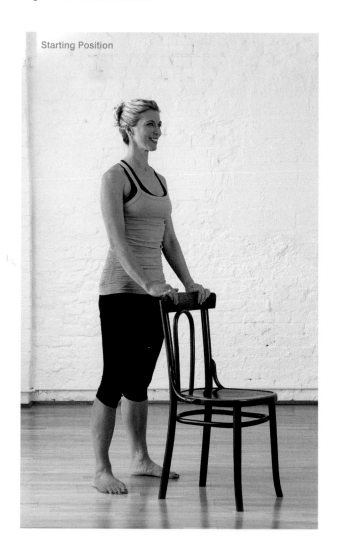

Starting Position

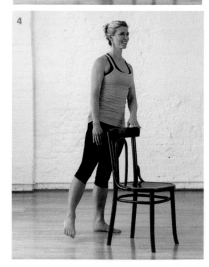

Action

Breathe normally throughout.

1 Transfer your weight on to the right foot, keeping the left toes on the floor, then transfer it back to the Starting Position before transferring it on to the left foot.

2 Progress the movement by lifting the left toes off the floor as you transfer your weight to the right foot, holding your weight there for a moment.

3 Repeat, transferring your weight to the left foot, lifting your right toes off the floor.

4 To challenge your balance further, place your hands more lightly on the chair or use just one hand.

Variation 1

Stand tall with the feet hip-width apart but keep both feet in contact with the floor while you transfer the weight.

Variation 2

Stand tall with a chair beside you and with feet in an offset Stance Position, one foot in front of the other (as shown top right). Place one hand on the chair. Transfer the weight forwards and backwards. Change legs and repeat.

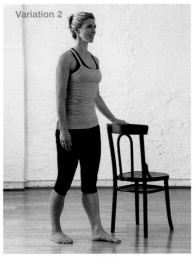

Variation 2

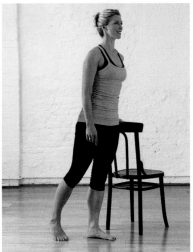

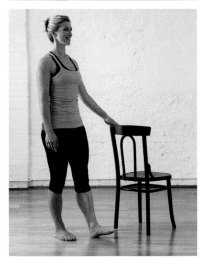

■ Avoid leaning with your upper body as you move; instead, stay lengthened and move your whole body on to one foot.

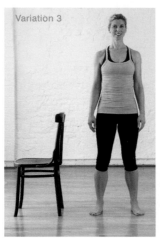 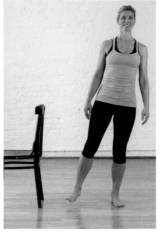 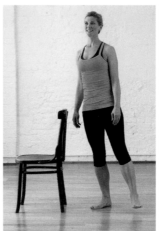 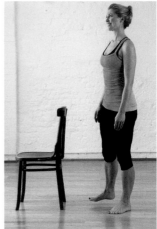

Variation 3

Stand tall, feet wider than hip-width apart and arms by your sides. Transfer your weight in a circle: shift the weight to the left and lift the right foot. As you lower the right foot and lift the left, rotate slightly to the left as if drawing a circle on the floor; keep the wider hip-width-apart position while moving. Once the circle is complete, repeat in the opposite direction.

Variation 4

Stand tall with one foot forwards, arms by your sides. Repeat the weight-transfer rotation as above.

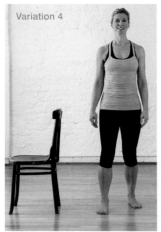 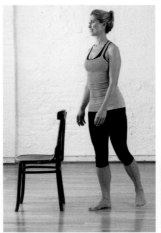 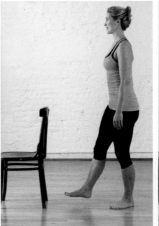 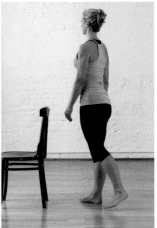

Tipping Point

This will challenge your Standing Alignment (p. 34) and thus improve your balance. Wear light, flexible, supportive, non-slip shoes if you wish.

Starting Position

Stand tall beside a sturdy chair (for emergencies), feet hip-width apart and arms by your sides. Use an appropriate level of core connection to control your alignment and movements.

Action

Breathe normally throughout.

1 Transfer the weight on to the balls of your feet, keeping your heels down.

2 Return to the Starting Position.

3 Transfer the weight on to your heels, keeping your toes down – the movement is coming from your ankle joints.

Repeat 6 times, then:

4 Lean forwards, lifting your heels and hold for a few seconds.

5 Return to the Starting Position, weight evenly distributed on your feet.

6 Transfer your weight slightly on to your heels, lifting your toes and holding for a few seconds.

7 Return to the Starting Position.

Repeat 6 times.

■ Keep your spine and pelvis in neutral, head in line with your spine.

■ Keep your legs straight, but not locked.

■ Keep your toes lengthened; do not grip with them. The movement occurs at the ankle joints.

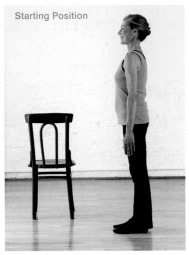
Starting Position

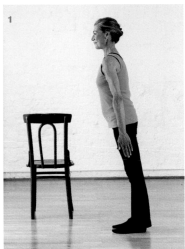
1

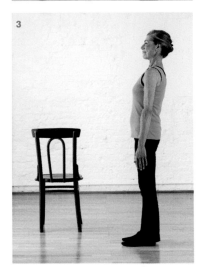
3

FUNCTIONAL REACHING

Reaching forwards and overhead can be taken for granted, but it is a skill we can lose as we age.

Reaching Forwards

Wear light, flexible, supportive, non-slip shoes if you wish.

Starting Position

Stand tall, feet hip-width apart and arms by your sides. Place a sturdy chair at arm's length in front of you.

Use an appropriate level of core connection to control your alignment and movements.

Action

Breathe normally throughout.

1 Reach forwards to the chair beyond your arm's length, lengthening your dominant arm forward. Keep your feet grounded.

2 Hinge at the hips to reach further forwards.

3 Return to the Starting Position.

Repeat 6 times, reaching with each arm.

Variation: stand tall with your feet in an offset position and repeat as above. The foot furthest forward should be an arm's length from the base of the chair.

Reaching Overhead

✳ Caution: take advice if you have shoulder problems. ✳

Starting Position

Stand tall beside a sturdy chair, feet hip-width apart and arms by your sides.

Use an appropriate level of core connection to control your alignment and movements

Action

Breathe normally throughout.

1 Reach one arm up and overhead, as if to reach a high shelf. While reaching, look at your fingers and keep the weight even on both feet with lengthened toes.

2 Return the arm to your side.

3 Repeat with the other arm.

Repeat 6 times.

✳ ■ Avoid locking your knees.

■ Try to maintain the distance between your ears and your shoulders as you reach.

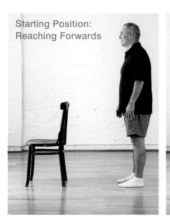
Starting Position: Reaching Forwards

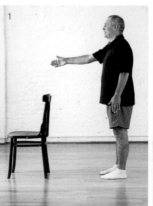
1

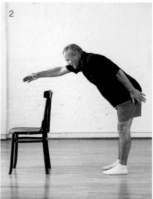
2

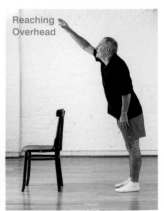
Reaching Overhead

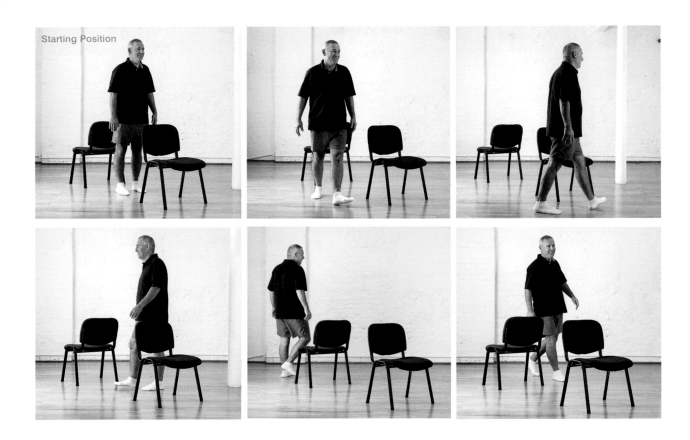

Starting Position

Figure of Eight

This challenges your ability to balance and change direction as you walk. Wear light, flexible, supportive, non-slip shoes if you wish.

✻ Take care if you have visual or ear problems. ✻

Starting Position

Stand tall between two sturdy chairs positioned about 60cm away from you as shown. Feet should be hip-width apart, your arms by your sides.

Use an appropriate level of core connection to control your alignment and movements.

Action

Breathe normally throughout.

Start walking, left foot forwards first, moving to the right and around the front chair. Continue walking around the chair and back towards the back chair, drawing an imaginary figure of eight with your steps. As you draw the eight, keep your feet hip-width apart.

Repeat 3 times, then change direction.

Variations

■ Try varying your walking speed.
■ Try walking with your feet more widely apart.
■ Try taking longer strides.

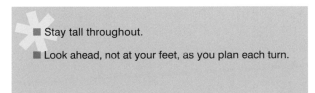

■ Stay tall throughout.

■ Look ahead, not at your feet, as you plan each turn.

FEET AND ANKLES

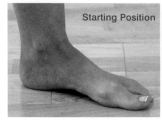
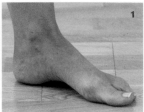

Starting Position

1

The foundation for the entire body, our feet are a highly complex combination of structures that serve to give us balance, stability, movement, carry our weight and act as shock absorbers. They accommodate to changes in our weight, and will adjust their shape and structure depending on the tasks being carried out. Acting in concert with the rest of the body during standing and movement, our feet play a leading role in our overall health and wellbeing.

If our foot structure is 'normal', correct signals are sent to the brain which, in turn, acts on these signals by maintaining good posture. Posture affects the health of all the weight-bearing joints and muscles in the body (the neck, back, hips, knees and ankles), and the efficiency of the feet when walking depends on the way in which these bones and joints move in relation to each other.

Efficient and pain-free function also depends greatly on the foot's angle to the leg and to the ground. If things do not work well in any of these areas, the joints become misaligned, leading to joint and muscle inflammation, causing pain throughout the body.

As well as pain, the effects of foot problems may show as instability, restricted movement or, in some cases, just fatigue. Even without pain, foot dysfunction can cause your whole body to overcompensate, which can then lead to back pain and even headaches, not to mention the emotional stress of discomfort and limitations on movement that can spread from the feet upwards.

Although the series of exercises that follows is specifically designed to promote healthy feet and ankles, you will, in fact, have been working on them throughout the book. This is because every time you exercise with your feet, ankles, knees and hips in good alignment, you are doing your feet and ankles a power of good. If you always remember to direct your knee over your second toe, you will be working your feet and ankles correctly.

Working the Arches

This exercise targets the arches of your feet. It is a subtle movement which is easy to miss, so please follow the directions carefully.

Starting Position

Sit tall or stand, so that the soles of your feet are on the floor. Have your legs hip-width apart and parallel.

Use an appropriate level of core connection to control your alignment and movements.

Action

Breathe normally throughout.

1 Keeping your toes long and ensuring they don't scrunch up, draw the base of the toes back towards the heels, thus increasing the arches.

2 Release the feet, returning them to a lengthened position.

Repeat up to 10 times, either working the feet separately or both together.

■ Avoid curling the toes; they should stay relaxed, keeping the action in the arches of the feet.

■ You may mimic the action with your hands, if that helps.

■ Ensure that your feet remain evenly planted on the floor and do not roll out or in.

■ Maintain good hip, knee and ankle alignment.

Mexican Wave

This exercise mobilises the joints of the foot and teaches you co-ordination and control of the feet.

Starting Position

Stand tall on the floor (not on your mat) and lengthen your spine into neutral. The legs are parallel and hip-width apart.

This exercise may also be performed sitting upright on a chair, feet grounded and hip-width apart on the floor. This is a useful position if you need your hands to help move your toes.

Action

Breathe normally throughout.

1 First, lift only your big toes off the floor, keeping the rest of your toes down. Then try to lift them off one at a time in sequence, until all the toes have peeled off the floor. If necessary, use your hands to help guide the movement and isolate the toes.

2 Replace your toes back down in sequence, starting with the little toe and spacing them out as widely as possible.

3 Reverse the movement: raise the little toes first, continuing one at a time to the big toe.

Repeat up to 5 times, either working the feet separately or both together.

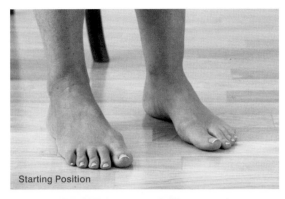
Starting Position

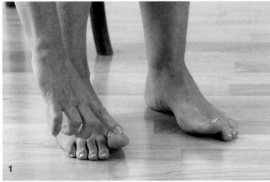
1

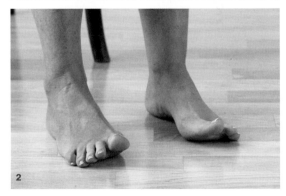
2

✱ ■ Maintain correct alignment of your leg: ensure that your foot, ankle and knee remain in line with your hip.

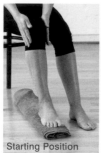
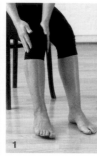
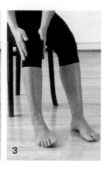

Starting Position   1   3

Eversion/Inversion

These are important actions for the health of your ankles and feet.

Starting Point

Sit tall on a sturdy chair, feet hip-width apart and hands on each side of one knee. If possible, rest your foot on a rolled-up towel. Otherwise, rest it on the floor.

Use an appropriate level of core connection to control your alignment and movements.

Action

Breathe normally throughout.

1 Slowly lift the outside border of the foot off the floor or towel. Maintain the arch height, the length of the toes and the knee alignment.

2 Return to the Starting Position.

Repeat 6 times, then:

3 Slowly lift the inside border of the foot off the floor or towel.

4 Return to the Starting Position.

Repeat 6 times.

> ■ Avoid moving the knee inwards/outwards along with the foot; the movement should initiate from the ankle, not the knee.
>
> ■ Maintain good hip, knee and ankle alignment.

Marching Feet

To improve plantar flexion (point) and dorsiflexion (flex) of the foot at the ankle. You can use what you learn here for Bridge With Marching Feet (p. 95).

Starting Position

Sit tall towards the front of a sturdy chair, feet hip-width apart and hands on your thighs.

Use an appropriate level of core connection to control your alignment and movements.

Action

Breathe normally throughout.

1 Simultaneously roll through both feet to lift the toes of the right foot and the heel of the left.

2 Then swap, rolling through the feet to lift the heel of the right foot and the toes of the left.

Repeat 10 times

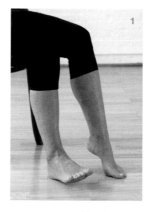
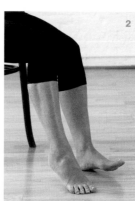

1   2

> ■ Check that your feet do not roll in or out as you march; as you lift your heel, send the front of the ankle directly forwards, and as you lift the toes, try not to swivel on the heel – stay central.
>
> ■ Watch for any unwanted movement in your spine; it should remain lengthened and still, your weight even on both sitting bones.

Ankle Circles

The goal of this exercise is to mobilise your ankle joints.

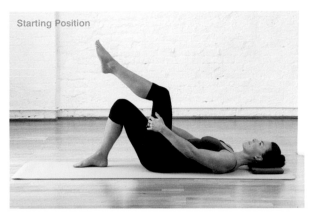

Starting Position

✱ Caution: take advice if you have an ankle injury. Take care not to flex your hip past 90 degrees if you have had a hip replacement in the last 6–12 weeks. ✱

Starting Position

Either: The Relaxation Position. With control, single-knee-fold and clasp your hands lightly behind your thigh (use a towel or scarf if you cannot reach). Lift your lower leg up slightly, so that your foot is higher than your knee.

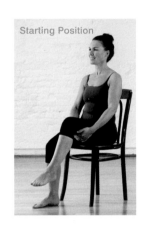

Starting Position

Or: Sit on a chair, fairly near the front. Lightly clasp your hands under your thigh or place a cushion there, so it is lifted slightly. Check that you are still sitting tall and your shoulders are open.

Use an appropriate level of core connection to control your alignment and movements.

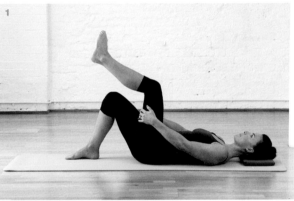

1

Action

Breathe normally.

1 Keeping your leg still, circle your raised foot outwards, moving from your ankle joint. Complete a full circle, trying to keep your foot and toes lengthened and free from tension.

2 Circle up to 5 times one way, then 5 times the other.

Repeat with the other ankle, up to 5 times in each direction.

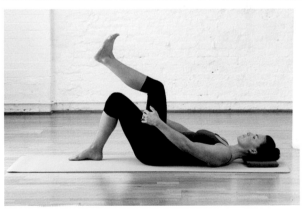

✱ ■ Avoid twisting your pelvis or side-bending your spine as you reach to hold your leg.

■ Keep your thigh and your shin bone still.

■ Try to keep your toes from being 'overactive'.

■ Attempt to create full and even circles.

■ Keep your chest and the front of your shoulders open and release any tension in your neck area.

HAND EXERCISES

In order for us to go about our daily activities easily, our hands need to have good:

■ mobility
■ strength
■ dexterity
■ co-ordination
■ sensation (in both static and dynamic tasks)
■ prehension (i.e. the tasks of grasping, holding and manipulating objects – functions described as grip and pinch).

These exercises help to develop and improve all of the above.

Ball Massage

Starting Position
Sit tall at a table and place each hand on a small ball.

Action
Move the ball forwards and backwards, right to left and vice versa, and in a circle.

■ Avoid moving the shoulders forwards and keep your spine and pelvis in neutral throughout.

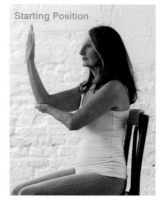
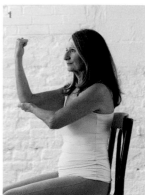

Starting Position   1

Make a Fist

Starting Position
Sit or stand tall with your feet hip-width apart, your right arm bent at the elbow to a 90-degree angle – forearm lengthening forwards and elbow under the shoulder. Support it with your left arm as shown. Your palm can be turned either upwards, inwards or downwards.

Action
1 Close the fingers in a fist with the thumb outside and then open them.

2 Repeat the above, holding the position for some seconds.

3 Repeat, making the fist tighter, then release.

Repeat the sequence 6 times, swapping arms.

Variation: if you found the movements painful, try placing your fingers over a medium soft ball and squeezing as you would to close the hand in a fist shape. Repeat the actions above. Once you've improved, use different-sized balls.

■ Adjust the position of your hand or arm if you feel any discomfort or pain.

■ Watch that the fingers close evenly.

Finger Actions

Starting Position
Sit or stand tall. Place your hands in front of your chest, arms bent at the elbows, palms facing away and fingers slightly open. Keep your shoulders open and relaxed.

Action 1: Play the Piano
1 With palms facing downwards and forearms horizontal to the ground, move your fingers up and down as if touching the keys of a piano.

2 Allow your forearms to move along the imaginary piano keyboard, the movement happening at the base of the knuckles, so your fingers remain long.

3 Repeat with the fingers curled.

Action 2: Play the Fingers
This one requires brain power too!

1 Start with the right thumb in contact with the left little finger and the left thumb in contact with the right little finger.

2 Move the right little finger outwards, then let the ring finger touch the left thumb, while simultaneously the right thumb moves inwards to touch the left middle finger.

3 Continue the movement as described to allow the thumbs to touch each finger of the opposite hand. This is a combination of wrist and finger movements.

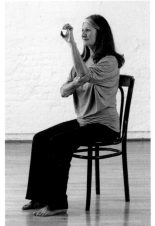 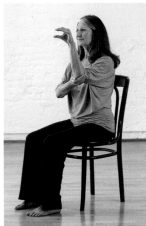

Duck

Starting Position
As opposite.

Action
Curl the fingers and the thumb inwards, towards the palm, then push them outwards, horizontally to the ground to form a horizontal V or a duck shadow. Keep your palm vertical throughout the movement.

Scrunch

Starting Position
Sit tall at a table, resting your forearms on it, palms down. Place two sheets of paper close to the fingers.

Action
Keeping the heel of the hands still, scrunch the paper. Repeat with different materials – a towel, a handkerchief or putty.

ADVANCED EXERCISES

The following exercises are for those who like an extra challenge.

Squat and Rotate

Practise this to improve and strengthen the hip, knee and ankle and encourage the stability of the lower body while moving the upper body.

Starting Position

Stand tall on the floor, feet hip-width apart. We have given you three different arm positions of increasing difficulty: arms lengthened down by your side; arms folded one over the other just at chest level; hands clasped behind your neck, elbows remaining within your peripheral vision.

Use an appropriate level of core connection to control your alignment and movements.

Action

1 Breathe in to prepare to move.

2 Breathe out as you bend your knees and hips, until your thighs are parallel to the floor.

3 Breathe in and maintain the position while you rotate your head, neck and spine towards the right.

4 Breathe out as you straighten both legs, keeping the spinal rotation.

5 Breathe in as you return to the Starting Position.

Repeat 5 times, alternating the rotation.

> ■ While rotating your head and spine, keep the pelvis in neutral and knees facing forwards.
>
> ■ Bend the knees and hips only as far as you can while keeping the pelvis and spine in neutral.

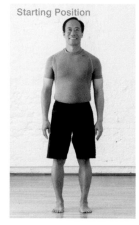

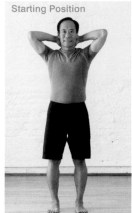

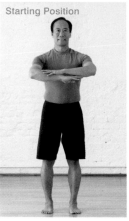

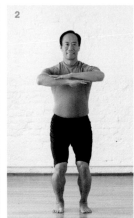

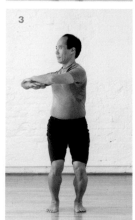

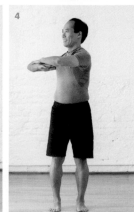

Variation: Lunge with Bow and Arrow (The Archer)

Here you combine two exercises, which makes it far more challenging.

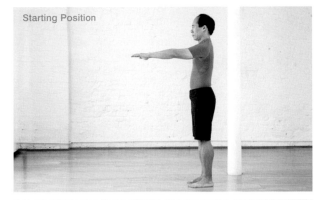

Starting Position

As for the Lunge (p. 96), but with your arms extended in front slightly lower than shoulder height and shoulder-width apart; palms down as for Bow and Arrow (p. 68).

Action

1 Breathe in as you step forward with your right foot, bending the right knee and hip to about 90-degree angles, while simultaneously extending the left hip and bending the left knee parallel to the floor.

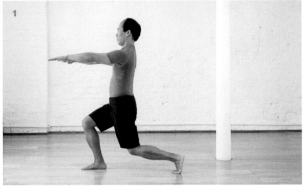

2 Breathe out as you bend the left elbow, drawing the arm towards the body and the left hand towards your shoulder. Simultaneously, rotate your head, neck and upper spine to the left.

3 Breathe in, holding the Lunge position; extend your left elbow and lengthen the arm away from your body. Lengthen the spine and encourage just a little more rotation (keeping the pelvis square to front).

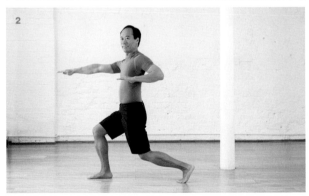

4 Breathe out as you rotate the spine back; keep the left arm straight.

5 Breathe in as you straighten the right leg and step back to return to the Starting Position.

Repeat 3 times on each side.

Variation: For an even more challenging version, lunge and rotate simultaneously.

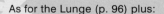

As for the Lunge (p. 96) plus:

■ In the final Archer position, feel the stretch through both arms. Reach through the front fingers, but take care not to deviate to one side.

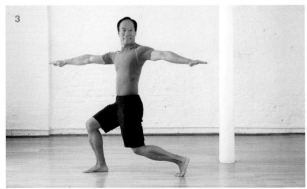

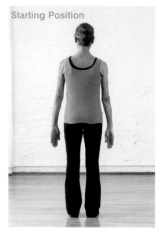
Starting Position
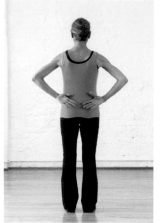
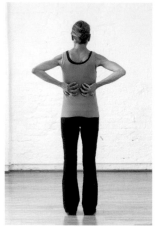
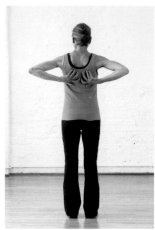

Back Scratch

To measure and improve your shoulder mobility.

Starting Position

Sit or stand tall, feet hip-width apart and arms by your sides.

Use an appropriate level of core connection to control your alignment and movements.

Action

Breathe normally throughout.

Reach with both hands behind your back, palms facing out, and reach up your back as far as possible. Touch the middle fingers, then, if comfortable, overlap them.

As you become more proficient, you may turn your palms to face your back to open your shoulders even more.

Repeat as comfortable.

■ Keep the alignment of the neck, spine and pelvis in neutral and still throughout.

■ Maintain the distance between shoulders and ears.

■ Avoid lifting or rolling the shoulders forwards.

Neck Scratch

To measure and improve shoulder mobility.

Starting Position

Sit or stand tall, feet hip-width apart and arms by your sides.

Use an appropriate level of core connection to control your alignment and movements.

Action

Breathe normally throughout.

Lift both arms to shoulder height, bend at the elbows and reach for the back of the neck, palms facing the head. Touch the middle fingers then, if comfortable, overlap them.

You may progress to lifting both arms overhead and repeat as above.

Repeat as comfortable.

■ Avoid bending forward and keep your head and neck in alignment.

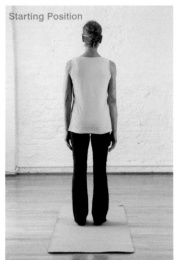

Starting Position

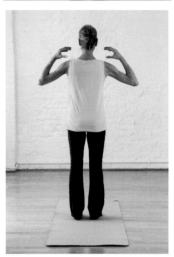

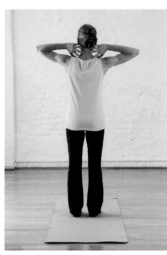

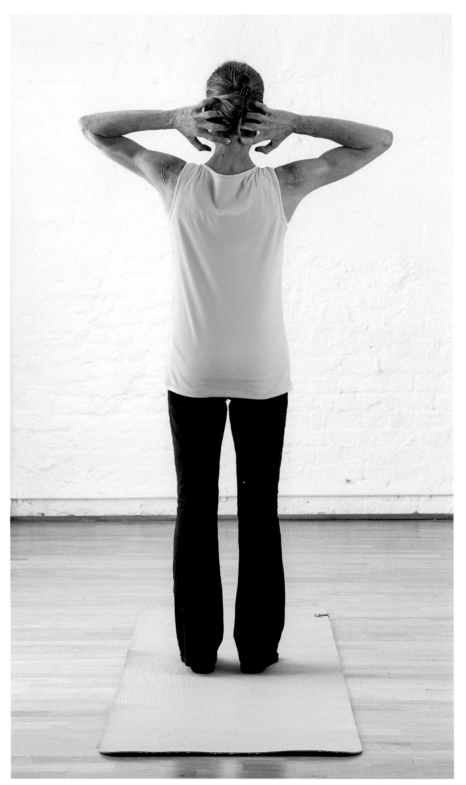

Main Exercise Programme

SUGGESTED WORKOUTS

The following workouts include exercises from the main Pilates for Life programme, the Fundamentals programme and a few from the Pilates for Health programme. They are about 45 minutes in length. If you are creating your own workouts you can choose exercises from anywhere in the book.

Workout One

- Starting Position: Relaxation Position (p. 23)
- Starfish (p. 48)
- Knee Rolls (p. 86)
- Spine Curls (p. 58)
- Arm Circles (p. 92)
- Oblique Curl-ups (p. 73)
- Bridge (p. 94)
- Hip Rolls (p. 66)
- Side-lying Bicycle (p. 117)
- Side-lying Bow and Arrow (p. 67)
- Dart (p. 108)
- Cobra Preparation (p. 61)
- Prone Knee Lifts (p. 49)
- Cat (p. 57)
- Rest Position (p. 62)
- Mexican Wave (p. 133)
- Working the Arches (p. 132)
- Triceps/Biceps (p. 106–107)
- Standing Dumb Waiter (p. 105)
- Side Reach (p. 70)
- Lunge (p. 96)
- Balance (p. 123)
- Tipping Point (p. 129)
- Tennis Ball Rising (p. 76)

Workout Two

- Starting Position: Standing on One Leg (p. 53)
- Weight Transfer (p. 126–29)
- Pilates Squat (p. 75)
- Relaxation Position (p. 23)
- Ribcage Closure (p. 47)
- Spine curls – Marching Feet Variation (p. 58)
- Curl-ups (p. 59)
- Zig-zags (p. 88)
- Chalk circles (p. 183)
- Side-lying Leg Lifts – with or without weights (p. 115)
- Cobra Preparation – Arm Slide Variation (p. 61)
- Full Star (p. 109)
- Full Table-top (p. 111)
- Rest Position (p. 62)
- Seated Pray (p. 113)
- Marching Feet (p. 134)
- Eversion/Inversion (p. 134)
- A vision exercise (pp. 78–81)
- Pelvic floor exercises: slow, quick and release (pp. 176–177)
- Standing Biceps Press (p. 106)
- Standing Side Stretch (p. 120)
- Travelling Lunge (p. 96)
- Figure of Eight (p. 131)
- Balance (p. 123)
- Sliding Down the Wall (p. 100)
- Roll Downs Against the Wall (p. 104)

Workout Three

- Starting Position: Relaxation Position (p. 23)
- Shoulder Drops (p. 46)
- Chin Tucks and Neck Rolls (p. 26)
- Windows (p. 91)
- Knee Rolls (p. 86)
- Single or Double Knee fold (pp. 44–45)
- Spine Curls (p. 58)
- Oblique Curl-ups (p. 73)
- Ankle Circles (p. 135)
- Diamond Press (p. 60)
- Cobra Preparation (p. 61)
- Cat (p. 57)
- Rest Position (p. 62)
- Oyster (p. 51)
- Side-lying Knee Cross-overs (p. 116)
- Side-lying Bow and Arrow (p. 67)
- Seated C-curve (p. 56
- Seated Thoracic Extension (p. 153)
- Seated Waist Twist (p. 64)
- A grip/dexterity exercise (pp. 136–137)
- Sliding Down the Wall with Ribcage Closure (p. 100)
- Lunge with Pick Up (p. 98)
- Functional Reaching (p. 130)
- Climb a Tree Preparation (p. 112)
- Bridge (p. 94) – add Knee Openings p. 43)
- Standing Star plus Side Reach (p. 119)
- Balance (p. 123)

Chair Workout

Just one example of a workout you can do whilst still in chair!

- Starting Position: Hand Press (p. 29)
- Scarf Breathing (p. 37)
- Pelvic floor exercises: slow, quick and release (pp. 176–177)
- Thumb Rolls (p. 77)
- Arm Swing (p. 114)
- The Nod (p. 27)
- Seated Waist Twist (p. 64)
- Side Reach (p. 70)
- Hip Hinge (p. 74)
- Seated Thoracic Extension (p. 153)
- Pray (p. 113)
- Dumb Waiter (p. 105)
- Working the Arches (p. 132)
- Marching Feet (p. 134)
- Seated Supported Wrist Exercises (p. 162–63)
- Biceps press (p. 106)
- Seated Knee Crosses (p. 161)
- Shoulder Boxes (p. 182)
- Bow and Arrow (p. 68)
- Seated Pillow Squeeze (p. 90)

PILATES FOR HEALTH

A study published in the *British Medical Journal* in 2013 showed just how influential exercise can be in extending lifespan. The research involved the analysis of 339,274 patients, comparing mortality rates among those prescribed medication for serious conditions with those enrolled in exercise programmes instead. Medication worked best for heart failure but, in all the other groups, exercise was as effective as drugs.

This study joins a huge body of evidence supporting the benefits of regular physical activity. Exercise has been shown to lower the risk of early death, help control weight and reduce the risk of heart disease, stroke, type-2 diabetes, depression, some types of cancer and a host of other conditions. It also lowers the risk of cognitive decline and hip fractures.

*Comparative effectiveness of exercise and drug interventions on mortality outcomes: metaepidemiological study

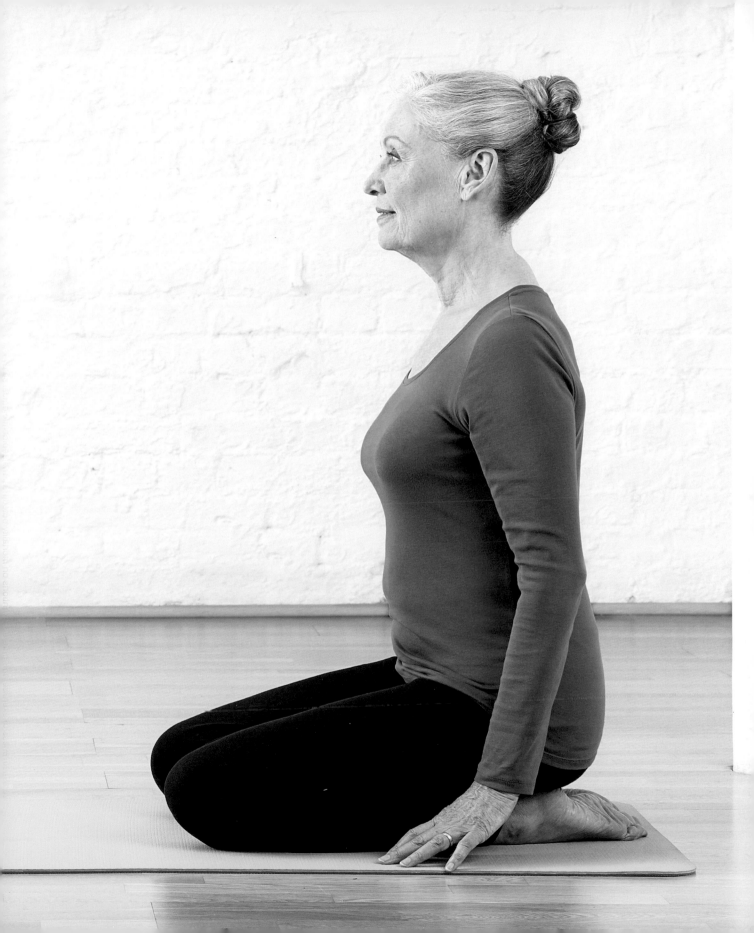

PILATES FOR BONE HEALTH

Osteoporosis has been termed 'the silent epidemic', affecting almost one in three women over the age of 50 in the UK. It is the gradual and silent loss of bone from our bodies, and happens in both men and women, but to varying degrees. In the UK it is diagnosed when there has been a loss of 25 per cent of normal bone density. Bone loss is expected as a normal part of the ageing process for many people, the inference being that there is little or nothing that can be done to stop or even slow down its progress. The World Health Organisation has stated that osteoporosis is 'entirely preventable', giving us reason to question what we see as inevitable, and to hope that we may be able to improve bone density.

Our bones are made up of a mixture of minerals, the most important being calcium, together with other trace elements. The bones in our body have an outer compact layer and an inner, less compact, centre. The latter has a honeycomb-like structure and is most affected by bone loss. When less calcium is absorbed in our bodies, struts in the honeycomb weaken, leading to micro fractures which can eventually develop into a full fracture, most commonly in the spine, hip and wrist.

'Strength training twice a week dramatically cuts the risk of fractures for postmenopausal women.'

There is a balance in the body between the bone-producing cells, the osteoblasts, and the cells that clear away dead bone, the osteoclasts. During our lives, this balance changes according to our needs and age. Factors such as diet, lack of exercise and stress may all contribute to the density of our bones. As we approach our mid-forties, our bone density can change for varied reasons, the main one in women being the menopause. A drop in oestrogen levels in the blood stream affects calcium absorption, resulting in an overall lessening of bone density. During the menopause women may lose up to 20 per cent of their bone density (Chopra 2002).

COMMON FRACTURE SITES

The most vulnerable areas are the wrist, hip, spine and ribs. Fractures of the wrist and hip may need hospital treatment but recovery is quick, whereas spinal fractures are more debilitating.

When bone has become less dense, fractures may occur in response to normal activities or to minor incidents. This history of a minor force causing a fracture is often the first sign that you may have osteoporosis, and will often lead to a diagnosis after the appropriate bone density scan. It is important to know your resulting 'T-score', which tells you how much bone you have lost: for example, a score of -2.5 means you have lost 25 per cent of your bone density. Appropriate exercises can then be recommended.

SAFE EXERCISE FOR OSTEOPOROSIS

Weight-bearing exercise involves activities which use free weights and the body's own weight against gravity. It is widely accepted that weight-bearing exercise is needed to increase bone density, but the good news is that the mechanical force exerted by the simple contraction of a muscle as it pulls on its bone of origin leads to an increase in bone production. In a 1994 article in the *Journal of the American Medical Association*, Miriam Nelson showed that strength training twice a week dramatically cuts the risk of fractures for postmenopausal women: after one year participants had gained bone in the hip and spine.

The more weight-bearing exercises we do, the more the bone-producing cells will be stimulated, so try to do regular 'aerobic' exercise appropriate for our age range, such as light jogging and moving jumps (under 50's), or brisk walking, for ten minutes at a time, as well as the Pilates programme recommended on p. 148.

Pilates can be immensely beneficial to anyone with osteoporosis as it offers a safe, systematic way of exercising which can stimulate bone production. Improving your balance, co-ordination, posture and core stability are high on the priority list for all Pilates sessions, and are essential in helping with bone-density conditions.

If you have been diagnosed with osteoporosis, you must check with your medical practitioner before you try Pilates. You will need to adapt your exercises as many traditional Pilates exercises may not be suitable for you. It is also beneficial to do more repetitions of certain exercises than would be normal in a generic Pilates class. Providing your technique is good, you may use heavier weights, as bones respond to a load greater than normal.

The list of exercises you will need to avoid is slightly controversial as the recommended guidelines in the UK differ from those in the US. The latter recommends only extension of the spine as being safe, and complete avoidance of trunk flexion, rotation and side flexion, which does not allow for much choice in exercise. We do not want you to be afraid to move, as this will compound the problem. UK guidelines are less rigid. The evidence against trunk flexion (that is Curl-ups, Roll Downs, and similar exercises) and also against combined flexion with rotation exercises is clear, so we will be avoiding these movements in this osteoporosis programme. Special care should be taken with side flexion and rotation exercises, but these may be done as long as sufficient support is provided and the movements are performed slowly and with proper control.

This gives us plenty of scope to maintain our range of movement, and increase it in some directions. It is also important to realise that Pilates will help to strengthen and improve the alignment around the joints, which is especially helpful for the spine. We will be focusing on back-extension exercises (such as the Dart and Diamond Press) in particular, as these are recognised as being hugely beneficial to spinal health. Top of our list will be promoting the length of your spine – think long and strong! We will also concentrate on exercises that target areas of the body which may be at risk. Improving your ability to balance is on the agenda too, since falls are the major cause of hip and wrist fractures.

Exercise for Osteopenia

Osteopenia is the precursor to osteoporosis. In simple terms, there is a smaller loss of bone density and because of this there are no real contra-indications to exercise except to be cautious with certain movements, such as unsupported trunk flexion and combined movements. Other than that, the advice is still to exercise regularly using weight-bearing work where we can, and maintain good alignment and flexibility whilst targeting specific areas of the body.

EXERCISE PROGRAMME FOR OSTEOPOROSIS

Our primary goals here are to:

■ use weight-bearing exercises to stimulate bone growth, targeting in particular the bones of the vulnerable sites (wrist, hips and spine)

■ improve your postural alignment to encourage length of the spine and reduce compressional forces

■ improve your balance and co-ordination to reduce the risk of falls.

■ target your anti-gravity muscles (in particular the deep core muscles and back extensors)

■ strengthen your muscles, so that they provide support around vulnerable sites

■ maintain your joint mobility

■ teach you the Hip Hinge (p. 74) to encourage you to bend from the hips and knees, rather than bending forwards from the spine

■ improve your relaxation and breathing techniques

■ improve your pelvic-floor control.

Recommended Exercises for Bone Health

The following are particularly beneficial for bone health, but please take medical advice if you have been diagnosed with osteoporosis:

■ Relaxation Position (p. 23)
■ Guided Relaxation (p. 180)
■ Pelvic-floor exercises (pp. 175–77)
■ Hand Press (p. 29)
■ Breathing exercises (pp. 168–69)
■ Shoulder Drops (p. 46)
■ Ribcage Closure (p. 47)
■ Oyster (p. 51)
■ Star Preparation (p. 49)
■ Standing On One Leg (p. 53)
■ Diamond Press (p. 60)
■ Cobra Preparation (p. 61)
■ Cobra Preparation with Arm Slide (p. 61)
■ Hip Hinge (p. 74)
■ Pilates Squat (p. 75)
■ Tennis Ball Rising (p. 76)
■ Thumb Rolls (p. 77)
■ Windows (p. 91)
■ Bridge and variations (pp. 94-95)
■ Lunge (p. 96)
■ Sliding Down the Wall (p. 100)
■ Wall Push-ups (p. 102)
■ Walking on the Wall Up and Down (p. 103)
■ Dumb Waiter (p. 105)
■ Biceps Press (p. 106)
■ Triceps (p. 107)
■ Dart (p. 108)
■ Full Star (p. 109)
■ Full Table-top (p. 111)
■ Side-lying Legs – Lift and Lower (p. 115)
■ Standing Balance Exercises (p. 123)

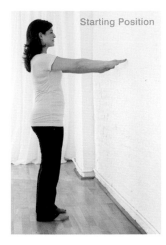
Starting Position

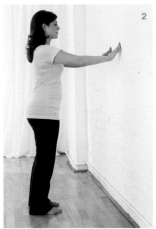
2

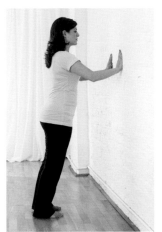

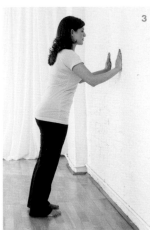
3

Wrist Loading

This exercise will help to promote bone density in the wrists. First you need to practise Wall Push-ups (p. 102). Once you are confident with them, you can try this more dynamic version.

✶ Caution: avoid if you have had a recent wrist fracture. You should feel no pain with this exercise. ✶

Starting Position

Stand tall, facing a wall, as far away as you need to be for only your fingertips to touch the wall. Your arms should be just less than shoulder-width apart, feet either hip-width apart or in Pilates Stance (p. 35). Now step a few centimetres further back from the wall.

Use an appropriate level of core connection to control your alignment and movements.

Action

1 Breathe in to prepare, and lengthen up through your spine.

2 Breathe out as you 'fall' towards the wall, keeping your body straight and using your hands to stop the fall.

3 Breathe in as you push yourself immediately away back to the Starting Position.

Repeat 12 times.

■ Keep your body long and strong; do not collapse in the middle. Your ribs should stay connected.

■ Bend your elbows downwards, but remember to stay open across your collarbones.

■ Keep your head and neck in line with the rest of your body.

■ You will have to hinge from your ankle joint to achieve the right movement.

Mini Bridge

This is a mini version of the Bridge on p. 94. You will have to be precise and only lift a few centimetres off the mat. The idea is that your spine moves as one piece; you do not move segmentally as for Spine Curls (p. 58).

✳ Caution: take advice if you have knee problems. ✳

Starting Position

Relaxation Position. Ensure that you do not have too thick a pillow or towel under your head. Less is better, so that you do not compress your neck as you lift.

Use an appropriate level of core connection to control your alignment and movements.

Action

1 Breathe in to prepare, and lengthen through the spine.

2 Breathe out as you lift your hips about 10cm off the mat, moving your spine in one piece. (You've swallowed that stick again!)

3 Breathe in as you hold this lengthened position.

4 Breathe out as you lower in one piece. Repeat 8 times.

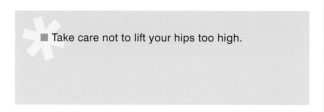

✳ ■ Take care not to lift your hips too high.

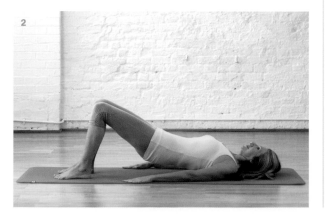

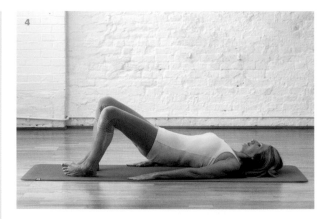

Mini Bridge plus Knee Openings

Moving on from the Mini Bridge, this requires you to take some of your weight on to one side, thus loading the hip joint.

✳ Caution: take advice if you have knee problems. ✳

Starting Position

As with Mini Bridge.

Use an appropriate level of core connection to control your alignment and movements.

Action

Follow Action points 1–3 for Mini Bridge, then:

4 Breathe out as you open one knee to the side as for Knee Openings (p. 43), keeping your pelvis lifted, still and stable, while your foot rolls to the outside edge.

5 Breathe in as you bring the leg back in line.

Repeat up to 6 times each side.

Mini Bridge plus Knee Folds

This is considerably harder than the Mini Bridge, as you take more of your weight on to your hip. Do not attempt this version until you are fully confident with the Mini Bridge, and stop if you cramp or feel any discomfort.

✳ Caution: take advice if you have knee or back problems. ✳

Starting Position
As before.

✳ ■ Maintain the length of both sides of the waist and keep the pelvis still as you move the leg.

Use an appropriate level of core connection to control your alignment and movements.

Action
Follow Action points 1–3 for Mini Bridge, then:

4 Breathe in and fold one knee in as for Knee Folds (p. 44); do not allow your hip to dip or pelvis to twist. Stay long and strong.

5 Breathe out as you lower the foot back to the Starting Position.

6 Breathe in as you fold the other knee in.

7 Breathe out as you lower your foot to the floor with control.

8 Breathe in as you lower back down to the mat in one piece with control.

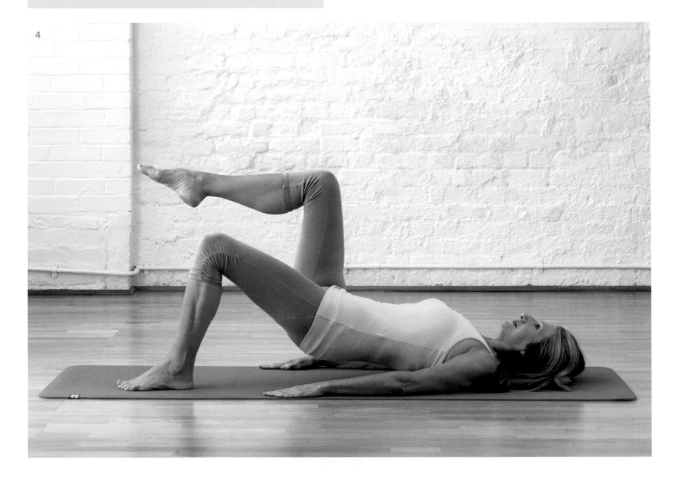

4

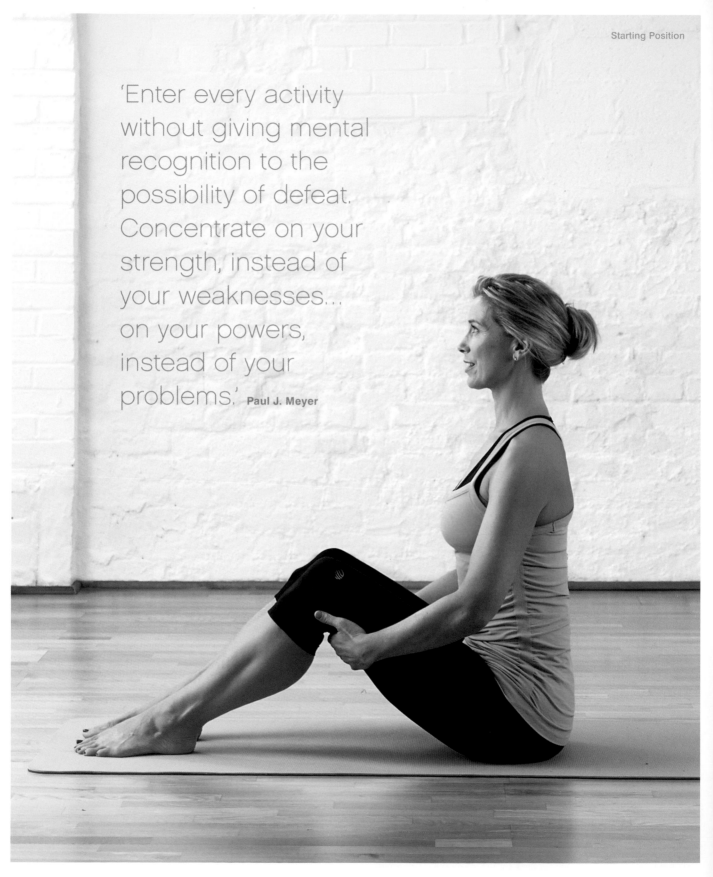

'Enter every activity without giving mental recognition to the possibility of defeat. Concentrate on your strength, instead of your weaknesses... on your powers, instead of your problems.' **Paul J. Meyer**

Seated Thoracic Extension

It is useful to be able to take what you have learned with Diamond Press and Cobra (pp. 60 and 61) into a seated position, as it means that throughout the day you can gently (and discreetly) take your upper back into extension and correct your posture. It is a subtle movement. If you are not convinced that your C-curve is elongated enough, leave it out and move from the neutral Starting Position into thoracic extension and back to neutral.

Starting Position

Sit tall on a mat with your knees bent, legs parallel and hip-width apart and the soles of your feet firmly grounded into the mat a comfortable distance away from the pelvis. Lightly hold the back of each thigh or, if you cannot reach, loop a towel around your thighs and hold the ends.

Alternatively, you may sit tall on a sturdy chair.

Use an appropriate level of core connection to control your alignment and movements.

Action

1 Breathe in as you lengthen your spine forwards into an elongated C-curve. Your shoulders should remain over your hips.

2 Breathe out as you lengthen back up into the neutral Starting Position, moving your pelvis and head simultaneously.

3 Breathe in and, starting with your head, sequentially extend your upper spine: head, neck and upper vertebrae; shine your breastbone forwards and up.

4 Breathe out as you lengthen and return the spine to the upright starting position.

Repeat up to 10 times.

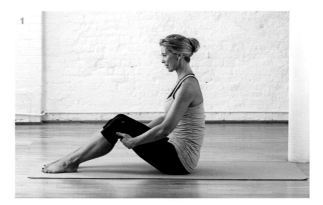

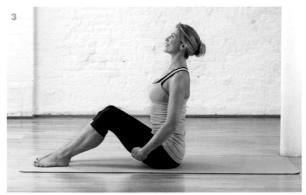

■ It is crucial that your C-curve is elongated and not collapsed.

■ Keep your shoulders down and open.

■ When you go into back extension, control your head and neck alignment; do not allow the head or neck to overextend.

■ Do not go back so far that you arch your lower back; it's the upper back we are targeting.

■ Keep your feet firmly planted on the mat/floor.

BACK EXTENSION, BACK EXTENSION AND MORE BACK EXTENSIONS

Starting Position

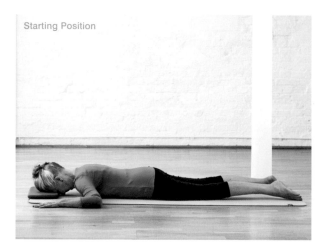

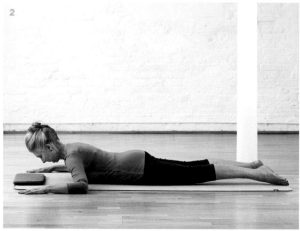

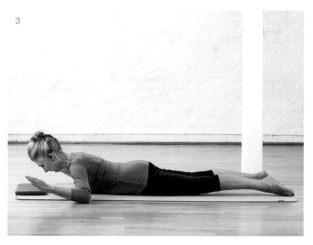

It is vitally important with osteoporosis to strengthen the spine and back muscles. The best way to do this is with back-extension exercises like Cobra Preparation (p. 61), Dart (p. 108), Full Star (p. 109) and Diamond Press (p. 60).

With slight adaptations, we can make the exercises even more effective. When you are doing your back extension, try adding an extra breath at the height of the movement.

With all the prone exercises, you may place a folded towel under your abdomen if it is more comfortable, as this will prevent your lower back going into extension; it is thoracic spine extension we are after.

Prone Windows /Cobra Prep variation

A challenging exercise, this is well worth the extra effort. Break it down and practise each stage in turn over several weeks or even months, if you need to. Start with Windows (p. 91) Cobra Preparation and Cobra Preparation with Arm Slide (p. 61), then add the forearm lift, then finally the arm extension and swimming action.

✱ Caution: take advice if you have back problems. Avoid if you have been diagnosed with stenosis of the spine. ✱

Starting Position

Prone, your forehead resting on the mat. (Use a folded towel if necessary.) Your legs should be straight, slightly wider than hip-width apart and slightly turned out from the hips. Bend your elbows and position your hands slightly wider than and above your shoulders, palms facing down. Ensure your shoulders are released and your collarbones are wide. Use a flat pillow or folded towel under your abdomen to help you maintain neutral.

Use an appropriate level of core connection to control your alignment and movements.

Action

1 Breathe in to prepare to move.

2 Breathe out as you begin to lengthen the front of the neck to roll and lift your head and then your chest off the mat. Your arms will begin to straighten slightly, but do not push into

them. Feel your lower ribs remaining in contact with the mat, but open your chest and focus on directing it forwards.

3 Breathe in as you stay lifted and lift just your forearms.

4 Breathe out as you straighten both arms; stay lifted.

5 Breathe in and bring both arms back down by your sides in a swimming-type movement, turning your palms inwards as you do so. Feel the crown of your head lengthening away.

6 Breathe out as you lengthen and lower your upper spine sequentially back down on to the mat.

7 Bring your arms back to the Starting Position.

Repeat up to 12 times.

Variation: this is slightly more challenging, as it requires you to stay with your back extended for a little longer.

Follow Action points 1–4 above, then move the arms out to the side in line with the shoulders before bending the elbows to bring them back to the starting position.

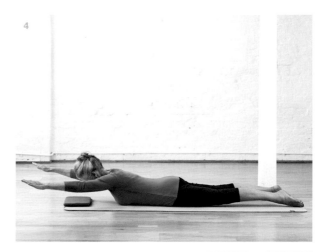

4

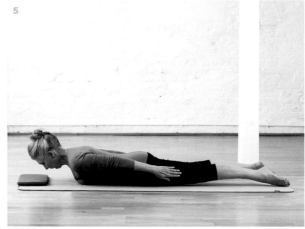

5

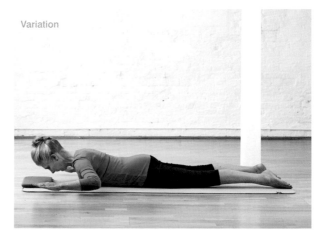

Variation

■ Initiate the back extension by lengthening and lifting your head first.

■ Keep your lower ribs in contact with the mat as you lift up, and try to maintain this position throughout.

■ As your forearms lift, try not to cheat by bending at the wrists!

■ Remember to turn your arms as you sweep them back down by your sides. Remember Arm Circles (p. 92) and Floating Arms (p. 52).

■ Keep your feet in contact with the mat throughout.

PILATES FOR JOINT HEALTH

Arthritis is a common condition which causes pain and inflammation within a joint (where two bone ends meet and provide movement). In the UK, around 10 million people have arthritis, which can affect people of all ages.

OSTEOARTHRITIS

Osteoarthritis, or OA, is described by some as a degenerative joint disease. Other definitions suggest that it is simply the natural result of ageing and wear and tear on the joints. However, younger people can be affected by osteoarthritis, too, often as a result of injury or another joint condition.

The first signs of osteoarthritis are normally pain and stiffness in the affected joint, which can progress to a reduced range of movement there. If the joint affected is the hip or knee, this will impact on walking. People with arthritis in the spine may find some daily activities, such as bending and lifting, more difficult. The pain and stiffness from an arthritic joint are more commonly experienced first thing in the morning and after being still in one position for any length of time.

As with the whole body, all structures within the joint are continually renewing themselves. OA is thought to develop when the body cannot keep up with the rate of repair needed to replace the cartilage cells in the joint (cartilage is the strong, smooth surface that lines the bones and allows joints to move with minimal friction and provides a degree of shock absorption). This leads to areas of unprotected bone being exposed, causing pain, stiffness, swelling and ultimately wearing away of the bony surface. The range of movement in the joint will also be affected and bony lumps, called osteophytes, may develop at the margins of the joint, which may or may not be painful.

Our joints are normally incredibly resilient, withstanding the strains and stresses we put on them throughout our lives. However, damage to a joint through injury can lead to arthritis, as can repetitive strains caused by work, and obesity, which increases the strain the joint experiences each day. There is an increased chance of developing osteoarthritis if you have a family history of the condition.

Joint replacements may be offered, but normally only when other therapies, such as physiotherapy, osteopathy, exercise and medication, have been tried. Whether you are offered surgery or not, it is important to keep the affected joints as mobile as possible with regular and safe exercise.

WHICH EXERCISES ARE BEST FOR OSTEOARTHRITIS?

Pilates can provide a safe and effective way of exercising for anyone who has OA, as it will help to improve the alignment of the joint or joints affected by strengthening the supporting muscles, and by maintaining and even improving ranges of movement. Some adaptations of the starting positions may be needed for certain exercises. For example, if kneeling is painful, place cushions under the knees. You may need to try alternative exercises which achieve a similar movement without aggravating your symptoms.

The most important things to think about are making sure you start the exercise in a good and well-aligned position so that the knees and feet are in line with the hips before you begin moving them. This will encourage the groups of muscles which work around each joint to work efficiently and keep each joint in its optimum position. It also encourages proper distribution of weight during daily activities which may encourage some repair of cartilage within the joint.

If you have osteoarthritis in your spine, it is important to improve the range of movement in areas which are stiff but not arthritic. Symptoms from the lower back may improve if the remainder of the spine is moving well. A classic area for stiffness is the thoracic spine – the middle-back area extending from below the neck to the lower ribs. A lifetime of bending over a desk can lead to stiffness here, which puts added strain on areas above or below. This may lead to arthritis developing or to existing symptoms worsening. Regular Pilates practice can ensure your whole spine is moving and you will begin to feel the benefit.

It is also important to strengthen your gluteal (buttock) muscles – the spine is much more likely to be positioned well over the pelvis and legs if you have really good, strong gluteal muscles. Society places great value on having a small bum, but small does not necessarily mean healthy! Make sure that, regardless of its size, yours is as strong as it should be.

So to summarise, our primary goals are to:

■ find the correct alignment of your affected joints
■ strengthen the muscles which support these joints
■ gently mobilise your joints
■ work in safe and supported positions
■ focus in particular on: articulating your spine, moving it segmentally, bone by bone, through flexion, extension and side rotation; mobilising the hip joints; toning the gluteal muscles; aligning the legs; strengthening the quadriceps; improving the grip and dexterity of the hands.

Rheumatoid Arthritis

Rheumatoid Arthritis is very different from OA. It is an 'auto-immune disease' in which the immune system attacks the body, producing inflammation of the joints with swelling, redness and stiffness. Over time, the repeated swelling can make the joint unstable. Joint alignment may be affected, making the joint vulnerable to injury. Symptoms normally appear on both sides of the body, and can be very debilitating over the years. The cause is not known and approximately 400,000 people in the UK are affected by it. If you have Rheumatoid Arthritis you must get expert advice before starting a new exercise regime. Pilates can help, but we would recommend one-to-one sessions with a qualified Pilates Teacher/ Medical Practitioner.

Recommended Exercises for Joint Health

The following exercises are particularly beneficial for joint health, but please take medical advice if you have been diagnosed with osteoarthritis. And always work within your comfort range:

■ Relaxation Position (p. 23)
■ Guided Relaxation (p. 180)
■ Chin Tucks & Neck Rolls (p. 26)
■ Hand Press (p. 29)
■ Breathing exercises (pp.168–69)
■ Leg Slides (p. 43)
■ Knee Openings (p. 43)
■ Single Knee Folds (p. 44)
■ Shoulder Drops (p. 46)
■ Ribcage Closure (p. 47)
■ Floating Arms (p. 52)
■ Starfish (p. 48)
■ Star Preparation (p. 49)
■ Prone Knee Lift (p. 49)
■ Oyster (p. 51)
■ Cat (p. 57)
■ Spine Curls (p. 58)
■ Diamond Press (p. 60)
■ Cobra Prep (p. 61)
■ Cobra Prep with Arm Slide (p. 61)
■ Waist Twist (p. 64)
■ Hip Rolls (p. 66)
■ Bow and Arrow (p. 67)
■ Side Reach (p. 70)
■ Hip Hinge (p. 74)
■ Pilates Squats (p. 75)
■ Tennis Ball Rising (p. 76)
■ Thumb Rolls (p. 77)
■ Knee Rolls and Prone

■ Knee Rolls (p. 86–87)
■ Zig-zags (p. 88)
■ Arm Circles (p. 92)
■ Windows (p. 91)
■ Sliding Down the Wall (p. 100)
■ Walking on the Wall Up and Down (p. 103)
■ Roll-downs (p. 104)
■ Dumb Waiter (p. 105)
■ Dart (p. 108)
■ Full Star (p. 109)
■ Lizard (p. 110)
■ Climb A Tree Prep (p. 112)
■ Seated Pillow Squeeze (p. 90)
■ Pray (p. 113)
■ Side-lying Knee Cross-overs (p. 116)
■ Side-lying Bicycle (p. 117)
■ Standing Balance (pp. 123–25)
■ Weight Transfer exercises (pp. 126–29)
■ Feet & Ankles exercises (pp. 132–35)
■ Seated Thoracic Extension (p. 153)
■ Long Stride (p. 124)
■ Functional Reaching (p. 130)
■ Figure of Eight (p. 131)

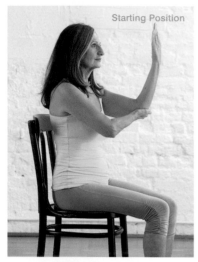

Starting Position

Finger Curls

These are like Roll Downs for the hands! The exercise will gently mobilise each joint.

Starting Position

Sit tall on a chair or on the mat and hold one arm out in front of you with the elbow bent at a 90 degree angle and the arm pointing upwards. You may support your 'working' arm with your other hand, or rest your elbow on a table. Be sure to check that your shoulders stay open and relaxed.

Action

Breathe normally throughout.

1 Curl just the top joints of your fingers down.

2 Then continue curling down each joint in turn.

Repeat 5 times with each hand.

Variation: Instead of curling each finger joint in turn, fold all the fingers down from the knuckles, then straighten up again. Repeat 5 times with each hand.

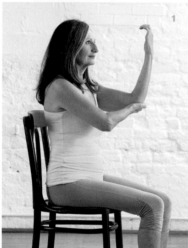

1

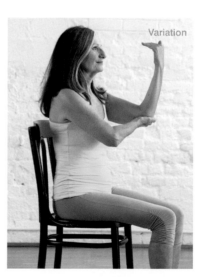

Variation

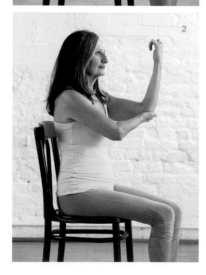

2

■ If you find this difficult, use your other hand to curl your fingers over.

Hide the Thumb

Starting Position
As opposite, but with your working hand resting palm up supported by your other hand.

Action
Breathe normally throughout.

1 Make a fist with your thumb on the inside.

2 Make a fist with your thumb on the outside.

Repeat 8 times with each hand.

Variation: once you have mastered the movement, have your palms facing each other and reach to touch the bottom of each finger with the tip of the thumb. Avoid closing the hand while moving the thumb.

■ Keep the wrist steady throughout.

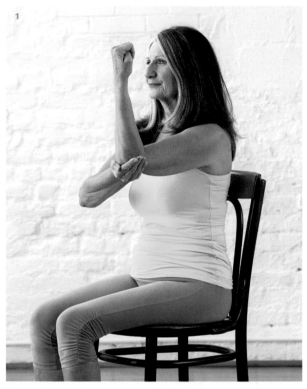

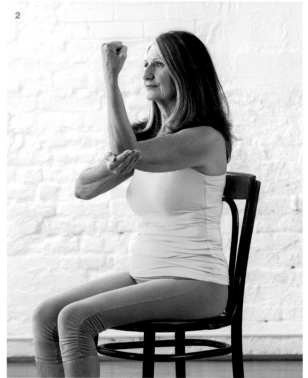

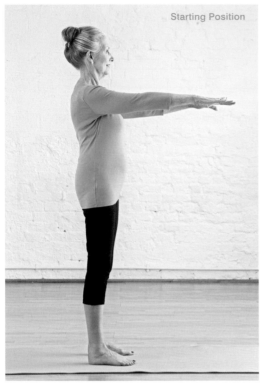

Starting Position

Standing Wrist Exercise

This is like Marching Feet (p. 134) but for wrist mobility. Keep good alignment throughout.

Starting Position

Stand tall with your feet hip-width apart. Reach your arms forwards to just below shoulder height, palms facing down.

Use an appropriate level of core connection to control your alignment and movements.

Action

Breathe normally throughout.

Move the right hand upwards from the wrist, simultaneously moving your left hand down.

Repeat 10 times.

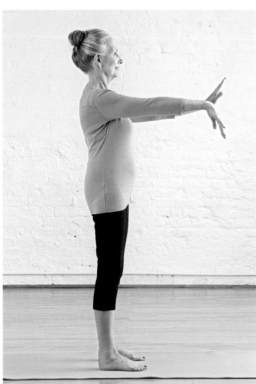

■ Stay open across your collarbones, maintaining the distance between your ears and your shoulders.

■ Keep standing tall, with your weight even on both feet.

Seated Knee Crosses

We are targeting the hip joints here, mobilising them gently. In normal circumstances, we would not advocate sitting with your legs crossed, but this is an exception! The key here is to stay upright and not sink down as your knee crosses over.

✱ Caution: take advice if you have had a hip replacement in the last 6–12 weeks. ✱

Starting Position

Sit tall in the middle of a sturdy chair, feet planted firmly hip-width apart (if your feet do not comfortably reach the floor, put a few books or a step under them). Check that your weight is evenly balanced on both your sitting bones.

Use an appropriate level of core connection to control your alignment and movements.

Action

1 Breathe in to prepare, and lengthen up through the spine.

2 Breathe out as you lift your right leg and cross it over your left leg, without twisting the pelvis.

3 Breathe in as you uncross your leg, still sitting tall.

4 Repeat with the other leg.

Repeat 8 times.

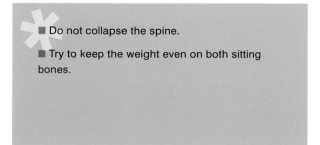

✱ ■ Do not collapse the spine.

■ Try to keep the weight even on both sitting bones.

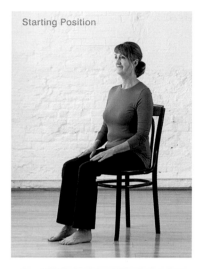

Starting Position

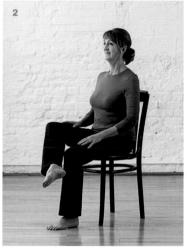

2

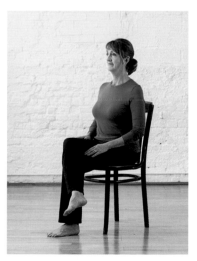

Seated Supported Wrist Exercises
These will help to improve your wrist mobility.

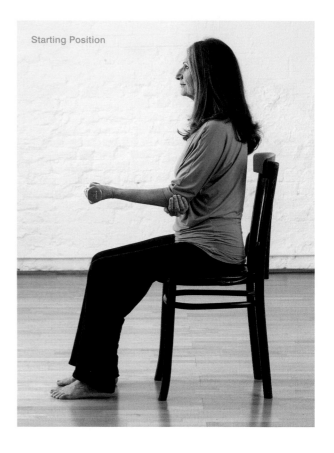

Starting Position

Starting Position
Sit tall on a sturdy chair with your feet hip-width apart. Place your right arm on the armrest with your hand off the edge of it (if there is no armrest, place your arm on a pillow or support it with your other arm). Make a fist, palm facing upwards. You may use a weight if you wish – start with very light weights and work up to using weights of about 1kg.

Use an appropriate level of core connection to control your alignment and movements.

Action
Breathe normally throughout.

1 Bend your hand towards you, moving upwards from the wrist.

2 Slowly return your hand to the Starting Position.

Repeat 10 times, then:

3 Make a fist with the palm facing down.

4 Bend your hand away from you, moving downwards from the wrist.

5 Slowly return your hand to a level position.

Repeat 10 times, then:

6 Make a fist with the palm facing in, thumb up.

7 Move your hand upwards.

8 Slowly return to the level position.

Repeat 10 times, then:

9 Place your arm by your side, palm facing in and thumb forwards.

10 Keeping your elbow still, move your wrist backwards.

11 Slowly return to the neutral position.

Repeat 10 times. Then repeat the above with your other hand.

> ✱ ■ Keep your forearm still as you do the wrist movements.
>
> ■ Stay lengthened in your spine; do not collapse.

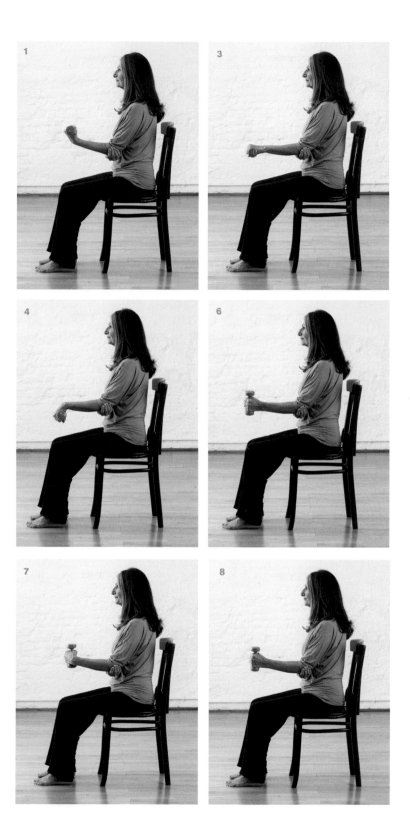

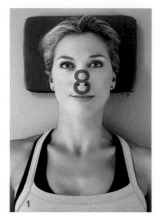

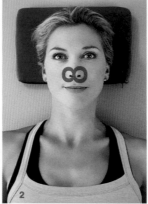

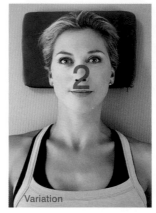

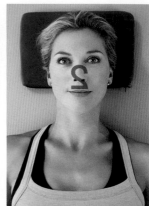

Variation

Nose Numbers

These oddly named exercises are a gentle and very relaxing way to mobilise the neck. You will be drawing the shape of different numbers with your nose – your head will of course follow the movement!

Start with the number eight. You need to imagine an upright figure eight for the first part of the exercise and one on its side for the second part. In both cases your nose starts where the two 'halves' of the eight cross.

✳ Caution: take advice if you have problems with dizziness. ✳

Starting Position

Relaxation Position with your arms lengthened by your sides. Your eyes may be open or closed.

Action

Breathe normally throughout.

1 Imagine an upright figure eight and trace the outline with your nose (your head comes along too!). It is a small smooth movement. Repeat 3 times, then change direction.

2 Now imagine the figure eight lying on its side. Trace again with your nose 3 times before changing direction.

3 Finish with a gentle Chin Tuck (p. 26), nodding the head forwards, drawing the chin down and lengthening the back of your neck.

4 Return to the Starting Position.

Variations: you can choose any number you wish. You can also add its mirror image. For example, with the number two.

■ The movements are very small and should feel comfortable. Be sure to perform them slowly and with control.

■ As you draw the chin down, ensure that the back of the head slides along the mat rather than simply pressing the back of the neck into the mat.

■ Try not to disturb the natural, neutral curves of your upper and lower back.

Knee Fold with Band/Scarf – Hip Flexion

Whereas with normal Knee Folds (p. 144) our focus is on pelvic stability, here it is on improving your hip flexion. You will need a stretch band or a long scarf.

✳ Caution: Don't take your hip beyond 90 degrees if you've had a hip replacement in the last 6–12 weeks. ✳

Starting Position
Relaxation Position. Fold one knee in and place the band across the front of the bent thigh. Hold the band with both hands. Keep the shoulders and collarbones wide and open.

Use an appropriate level of core connection to control your alignment and movements.

Action

1 Breathe in to prepare your body to move.

2 Breathe out as you press your leg towards you into the band, increasing your hip flexion.

3 Breathe in as you relax, but do not collapse!

Repeat 10 times with both legs.

> ✳ ■ Keep your pelvis and spine still and centred throughout; do not lose neutral.
>
> ■ Keep your leg directly in line with your hip joint.

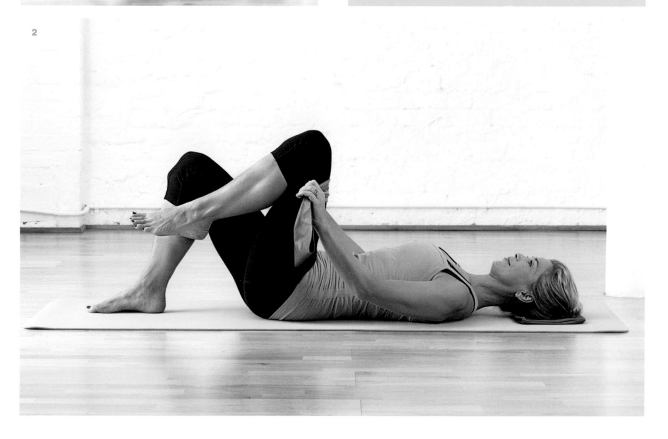

Starting Position

2

PILATES FOR RESPIRATORY HEALTH

As we age, we may experience changes that affect our lungs, which can then limit the activities of daily life. These changes may be due to the late onset of asthma, or the development of chronic bronchitis or emphysema, both of which can, in turn, lead to the more serious chronic obstructive pulmonary disease (COPD). Problems with our lungs can also occur as a result of heart disease.

ASTHMA

Asthma may start in childhood, as it did with Joseph Pilates, but many people develop it in later life, and this is known as adult-onset asthma. It may be triggered by allergies such as pollen, house dust mites, perfume, chemical irritants or smoke. It can also develop after illnesses such as colds and flu, and has even been linked to depression. The irritants within the airways cause an inflammatory reaction which tightens the tubes and thereby narrows them, making breathing more difficult.

The commonest symptoms of asthma are shortness of breath, wheezing, coughing and a feeling of tightness in the chest, but asthma can be harder to diagnose in adults as the symptoms are so similar to other chest conditions such as bronchitis and emphysema.

On the whole, asthma can be very well controlled by the use of medication and inhalers, and sufferers are encouraged to lead an active and healthy lifestyle. Many people are put off exercising because they believe it might worsen their condition, but research has found that exercise will benefit most sufferers. If in doubt, as always, consult your GP before you start a new exercise regime.

People with asthma (or other respiratory problems) tend to breathe more shallowly, using the upper chest. This is a less efficient way to breathe as it tends to draw air only into the upper areas of the lungs. Pilates is a safe way to begin exercising if you have asthma and will teach you how to breathe more deeply and efficiently, taking the air down into the base and sides of your lungs. A slower and deeper breathing pattern can help by increasing lung capacity and, therefore, their overall efficiency. Another benefit is that it helps to mobilise the thoracic area of the back (the middle area of the spine around the ribcage). People with breathing problems tend to get stiffer in this region partly because they are not breathing as deeply as normal, and this shallow pattern of breathing involves less movement of the ribcage. It can then become harder to take a deeper breath, simply because the rib joints with the spine do not move as well and so are less able to expand the lung space and draw in more air.

Caution: always have your inhaler nearby when you exercise.

BRONCHITIS/CHRONIC BRONCHITIS

Bronchitis can cause breathlessness and an altered breathing pattern. It is a result of inflammation in the tubes of the lungs, leading to increased production of mucus, causing a chronic cough. It may be diagnosed when there have been repeated bouts of chest infections, often beginning with a simple cold.

Causes of bronchitis, whether acute or chronic, are as you might expect: smoking, repeated exposure to chemical irritants, and viral infections. You need to do as much as possible to keep away from such irritants, which can reduce the number of acute attacks. Treatment for bronchitis may include medication to combat infection, inhalers to open the airways and exercise.

EMPHYSEMA

Emphysema is relatively common, often resulting from years of smoking or from being exposed to irritants. The lungs tend to lose their natural elasticity and are less able to fully expel the air breathed in. This leads to a feeling of breathlessness due to the air trapped in the lungs, which can be very debilitating. In fact, Joseph Pilates died of it in 1967, having smoked cigars for years and been exposed to smoke following a fire in his New York studio.

Learning to relax and breathe at a gentler but deeper rate, without forcing the air out, which is in line with the breathing patterns advocated in Pilates, can be very beneficial.

CHRONIC OBSTRUCTIVE PULMONARY DISEASE (COPD)

COPD is much more serious than bronchitis and may be life threatening. It can also be caused by other respiratory diseases, such as asthma. It is characterised by shortness of breath caused by the inability to draw enough air into the lungs and then to oxygenate the body. A chronic cough develops and there may be associated wheezing. There is the potential to develop secondary problems because not enough oxygen is being brought to the muscles of the body which may then become weak, affecting overall strength and stamina required to perform normal daily tasks.

Mild COPD can be helped by Pilates, but only under supervision and with advice from your doctor. You may find that the upright exercises are more beneficial initially.

Caution: if you have been diagnosed with moderate to severe COPD, you should only exercise under the care of a pulmonary rehabilitation team and your medical consultant.

'Learning to relax and breathe at a gentler but deeper rate can be very beneficial.'

EXERCISING FOR RESPIRATORY HEALTH

If you have been diagnosed with asthma, chronic bronchitis or emphysema, you will need medical permission to exercise. Stay mindful of the impact on your breathing pattern while you do the exercises and do not exert yourself to the point of breathlessness. You should also ensure that you keep all the appropriate medications/inhalers close by.

So to summarise, our primary goals here are to:
■ encourage a more relaxed, rhythmic and efficient way of breathing
■ improve the mobility of your spine and ribs, so that more air is drawn in.

Remember, as always, to think about good alignment before you try any breathing exercise, as efficient breathing relies on good posture. It is very difficult to breathe well if your ribs are compressed and your main breathing muscle – your diaphragm – is restricted.

We want to focus on a deeper, more rhythmic way of breathing that encourages the diaphragm to move up and down more which, in turn, allows the thoracic cavity to expand properly. A full inhalation followed by a deep exhalation helps increase your capacity to inhale new fresh air.

BREATHING EXERCISES

Here are a selection of breathing exercises in different positions, in which you use your hands and awareness techniques to help improve your breathing.

Repeat each exercise as many times as necessary for your breathing to become calmer, fuller and more rhythmic.

Scarf Breathing

Please revisit this exercise (p. 36) as it is fundamental to a good breathing technique. Scarf Breathing may be done seated or standing.

More breathing exercises

■ Relaxation Position. Wrap your arms around the front and sides of your lower ribs, keeping your shoulders and arms relaxed. Inhale and feel the expansion of the back and the sides of the ribs with your arms. Exhale and gently hug your lower ribcage as the lungs empty and allow the ribs to release fully.

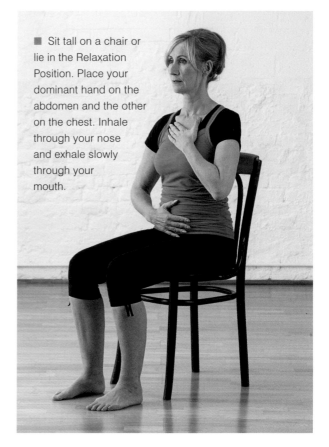

■ Sit tall on a chair or lie in the Relaxation Position. Place your dominant hand on the abdomen and the other on the chest. Inhale through your nose and exhale slowly through your mouth.

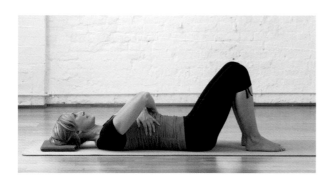

■ Relaxation Position. Place your hands on your abdomen to feel the movement of the diaphragm. Close your eyes, inhale through the nose (try to be aware of the expansion of the abdomen), hold your breath for up to 5 seconds, then breathe out fully, focusing on the movement of the abdomen.

■ Relaxation Position, placing your hands on your chest. Breathe in; be aware of the expansion of the ribs, then hold your breath for up to 5 seconds and exhale.

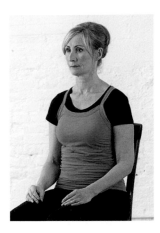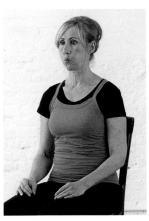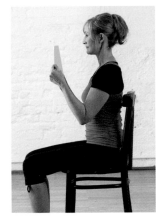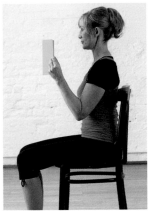

■ Sit tall on a chair. Blow air into an imaginary balloon and be aware of its expansion and contraction during your inhalation and exhalation.

■ Start in a seated position, sitting tall (when you are more proficient you can try this in the Relaxation Position). Hold a very light sheet of paper in front of your mouth. Be aware of the movement of the paper as you breathe in and as you breathe out through your mouth, and observe the movement of the sheet during strong exhalation and inhalation.

■ Sit tall on a mat or chair. Breathe in to a count of 3 seconds, hold your breath for a count of 3 seconds and breathe out for a count of 5 seconds. As you become accustomed to this pattern of breathing you may progress to 4, 4, 6, then 5, 5, 7 and so on.

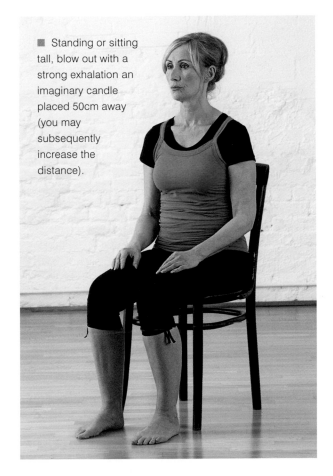

■ Standing or sitting tall, blow out with a strong exhalation an imaginary candle placed 50cm away (you may subsequently increase the distance).

■ Standing tall, breathe in as you take 3 steps forwards. Breathe out as you take 3 steps back. Then reverse the breathing. As you become accustomed to this pattern of breathing and walking, you can take 4 steps, 5 steps, etc. If you find it easier, increase the number of steps while breathing out and decrease the number of steps when you breathe in.

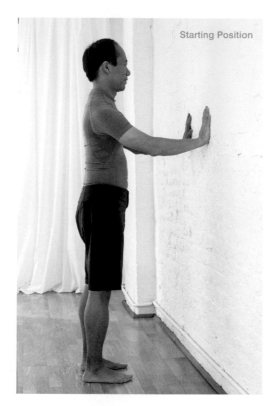

Starting Position

Thoracic Stretch Against the Wall
This stretch has been designed to help open out your ribs and back.

✳ Caution: take advice if you have back problems. ✳

Starting Position
Stand tall facing a wall about 60cm away. Lean both hands on the wall, no higher than shoulder height and just wider than shoulder-width apart.

Use an appropriate level of core connection to control your alignment and movements.

Action
1 Breathe in to prepare to move.

2 Breathe out as you slowly lower your head and upper body forwards through your arms until you feel a stretch in the upper back, without dropping your head below your arms.

3 Breathe in to the back of your ribs; enjoy the space the stretch has created.

4 Breathe out as, with control, you return your upper body to upright.

Repeat 5 times.

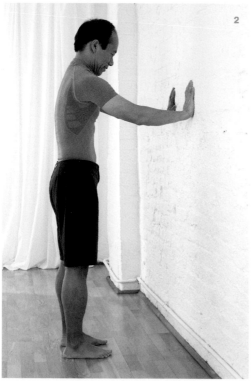

2

✳ ■ Always keep a connection into the centre of your body as this will keep your lumbar spine in a neutral and safe position.

Standing Thoracic Rotation at the Wall

Another exercise to mobilise your spine and ribcage. You will need to remember everything you learned in Waist Twists (p. 64).

Starting Position

Stand tall, side-on, about 45cm away from a wall, your feet hip-width apart and your arms held out in front of you, just below shoulder height.

Use an appropriate level of core connection to control your alignment and movements.

Action

1 Breathe in to prepare to move.

2 Breathe out as you turn your head, neck and upper body towards the wall, stretching your arms out to touch the wall behind you. Keep your pelvis still, facing front.

3 Breathe in and lengthen up through the spine. Increase the rotation if you can.

4 Breathe out and return your upper body, neck and head to face the front.

Repeat 5 times slowly before turning round to face the other way and repeating.

✳ Other Recommended Exercises for Respiratory Health

■ Relaxation Position (p. 23)
■ Guided Relaxation (p. 180)
■ Starfish (try doing this at half the speed with a slower breathing pattern) (p. 48)
■ Ribcage Closure (p. 47)
■ Cat (p. 57)
■ Side Reach with Breathing (p. 72)
■ Bow and Arrow – Seated and Side-lying (p. 67–8)
■ Chalk Circles (p. 183)
■ Dumb Waiter (p. 105)

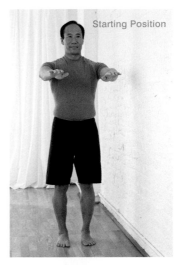

Starting Position

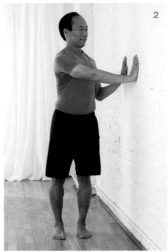

2

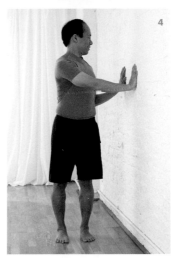

4

PILATES FOR HEART HEALTH

HEART HEALTH

Cardiovascular disease is the general term used to group together conditions involving the heart and the circulation. This includes heart attacks and angina (known together as coronary heart disease), as well as problems with the blood supply to the legs (known as Peripheral Vascular Disease).

The heart needs a strong blood supply to keep it healthy and when there are problems with this blood supply we can experience heart disease. The blood vessels which carry the blood to and away from the heart need to be healthy with a clear passage for the flow of blood through them. Over time, the walls of these vessels can become narrowed by calcium deposits, fat and inflammatory cells, potentially reducing the blood flow to the heart. Sometimes a clot may form and block the blood vessel completely.

Causes of coronary heart disease are mostly linked to lifestyle factors, such as smoking, drinking, obesity, a high-fat diet, lack of exercise and stress. As such, it is largely preventable.

The symptoms of heart disease are traditionally known to be tightness or pain in the chest, difficulty breathing, pain radiating to the jaw or down the left arm and sweating. However, there is mounting evidence to suggest that these symptoms are typical of what is now known as the 'male pattern heart attack' and the symptoms experienced by women can be very different. Women can have little or no chest pain, experiencing only extreme fatigue, back pain, vomiting and sometimes abdominal pain, and only occasionally central chest pain. Consequently, it appears more women are dying from atypical heart attacks than men, according to Dr. C Noel Bairey Merz, Professor of Medicine at Cedars–Sinai Heart Institute.

MEDICAL TREATMENT FOR CARDIOVASCULAR DISEASE

Angina is treated with medication to lower blood pressure, among other things, and a controlled exercise programme, including gentle cardiovascular exercise. This programme will be designed by medical experts, so if you have angina please always consult your doctor or consultant before trying any new form of exercise. Special care must also be taken if your angina is not stable, that is, if your symptoms are not well controlled by medication.

If you have had a heart attack you may have been given an angioplasty or even a coronary bypass operation. These procedures, which restore good blood flow to the heart, are not in themselves a cure, and long-term lifestyle changes need to be undertaken as well. Pilates can be valuable here, but only with medical clearance. After you have completed your cardiac rehabilitation programme and had your sign-off, recovery may seem slow, as your confidence in your own body may have been greatly shaken after experiencing a heart attack. Exercise has been shown to be one of the major factors in improving health after such an incident.

PERIPHERAL VASCULAR DISEASE (PVD)

This condition affects the blood flow to the legs due again to a build-up of fatty deposits in the walls of the arteries, which restricts the amount of blood flowing to the legs. The symptoms are pain and aching in the legs, primarily during walking and exercise (sometimes confused with similar symptoms from spinal stenosis). The condition is very much age-related, but the biggest causes are the same as those for heart disease, namely lifestyle choices.

'To maintain the health of your heart you need to include aerobic activities in your exercise regime.'

Treatment is with medication and, more importantly, changing the way we live. Sadly, there is a strong link between PVD and developing more serious heart disease and, in some circumstances, it can lead to amputation of the foot or leg.

Suitable Pilates exercises are valuable here, but must be done with medical permission.

Caution: always leave short periods of rest between exercises to allow the muscles to recover if blood flow is restricted.

EXERCISING FOR HEART HEALTH

Pilates is not a cardiovascular exercise. To maintain the health of your heart you will need to include some additional aerobic activities in your exercise regime. If you have a heart condition, you should take medical advice as to which aerobic activities are appropriate for you. You should also take into account any other conditions you may have.

Exercise guidelines
According to NHS guidelines, to stay healthy and prevent heart disease, adults should try to be active daily and do:

■ at least 150 minutes (2 hours and 30 minutes) of moderate-intensity aerobic activity such as cycling or fast walking every week
or
■ 75 minutes (1 hour and 15 minutes) of vigorous-intensity aerobic activity such as running or a game of singles tennis every week
or
■ An equivalent mix of moderate- and vigorous-intensity aerobic activity every week (for example two 30-minute runs plus 30 minutes of fast walking).

Moderate-intensity activity will raise your heart rate and make you breathe faster and feel warmer. One indication that you're working at a moderate intensity is if you can still talk, but you can't sing the words to a song.

Vigorous-intensity aerobic activity means you're breathing hard and fast, and your heart rate has gone up quite a bit. If you're working at this level, you won't be able to say more than a few words without pausing for a breath.

It seems that any activity which makes you break into a sweat, even gardening or household chores, will, if done regularly, lessen your chances of dying prematurely.

In addition to aerobic activity, all healthy adults should include muscle-strengthening activities on two or more days a week that work all major muscle groups (legs, hips, back, abdomen, chest, shoulders and arms). Your Pilates practice will contribute to this.

EXERCISING WITH DIABETES

If you have been diagnosed with diabetes – either type 1 or type 2 – you will know that physical exercise is recommended to help control your symptoms. In addition to all the well-known benefits, regular exercise can help improve your blood-sugar levels, as well as increase the levels of 'good' cholesterol in your bloodstream. It can also lower your blood pressure. If you have had diabetes for many years, you may be experiencing a change in the sensation to your feet, making walking and balance more difficult. As we have seen, many Pilates exercises can improve your balance, which helps to prevent falls.

Always be aware of your blood-sugar levels before and after exercising. If you are exercising for more than an hour it may be even more important that you monitor your levels during exercise and have whatever you need with you in case you begin to feel unwell.

EXERCISING WITH HIGH BLOOD PRESSURE

If you have been diagnosed with high blood pressure, you may be on medication to control it, as well as going for regular blood-pressure checks.

Exercising is recommended to help lower and control high blood pressure and Pilates is ideal, as the gentle and relaxed breathing and slow movements, can help to lower stress levels and therefore blood pressure over time. Intensive bouts of exercise are not recommended, as this will increase blood pressure and put unwanted strain on the heart.

The most important thing to remember when doing Pilates is not to hold your breath, which can raise your blood pressure very quickly. The slow and rhythmic breathing patterns taught in Pilates are therefore very valuable.

Caution: if your blood pressure is high, your doctor may prefer that you use medication to lower it before you start an exercise regime, so do consult your GP first.

'Ageing has a wonderful beauty and we should respect that.' **Eartha Kitt**

PILATES FOR WOMEN'S AND MEN'S HEALTH

We promised you a chapter devoted to the health of the pelvic floor and here it is!

Your pelvic-floor muscles span the base of your pelvis and work to help keep all your pelvic organs in place (preventing prolapses), to tightly close your bladder and bowel (preventing incontinence) and to help with sex. If your pelvic-floor muscles become weak or if they do not work in the right way at the right time, then you are likely to have problems; they need to be exercised regularly to keep them toned, just as you would work other muscles.

Pelvic-floor muscle problems can affect people of all ages, but the prevalence of incontinence increases with age in both sexes – it is not just a women's problem. Pregnancy, childbirth and, later in life, the menopause are obvious risk factors for women, while being overweight, smoking and being constipated are contributory factors for both sexes.

Symptoms of pelvic-floor muscle problems are varied and may include any of the following:

■ leakage of urine when coughing, sneezing, laughing, straining, lifting or jumping; for men, standing up from sitting or bending over may also cause leakage
■ an urgent feeling of needing to go to the toilet, possibly leaking on the way – this is known as urge incontinence
■ anal incontinence – an inability to prevent passing of wind or faeces
■ a prolapse, which may be felt as something bulging or a dragging sensation in this area; women may suffer from various types of prolapse which occur when the tissues supporting a pelvic organ are no longer able to hold it in place
■ reduced sensation during sex
■ overflow incontinence in men: this is the seepage of urine when the prostate gland becomes enlarged in men, blocking the normal flow of urine through the urethra; overflow may also result from nerve damage
■ erectile dysfunction
■ following a prostatectomy – incontinence, frequency of urinating, erectile dysfunction.

'Our bodies are gardens to which our wills are gardeners.' **William Shakespeare**

If you suffer any of these symptoms, do consult your doctor as there are specialist physiotherapists who can help (see Further Information, p. 217).

PELVIC-FLOOR EXERCISES FOR MEN AND WOMEN

To get the best results it is very important that you work the right muscles in the right way. It is very easy to get it wrong. This is why specialist help is always best, if possible, although at the end of the day you will have to do the exercises yourself.

You will need to do different types of exercises as pelvic-floor muscles have different types of fibres (slow-twitch and fast-twitch fibre) and we need to work both.

To locate the right muscles we need to revisit the Wind Zip.

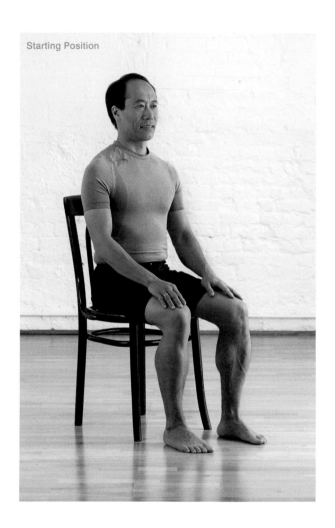
Starting Position

The Wind Zip Revisited

In this instance we are looking to locate and strengthen the pelvic-floor muscles rather than connect to your core. Once you have found the muscles, we can try Slow and Quick Zips.

Starting Position

Either: Upright on a chair with your feet on the floor, hip-width apart, making sure that your weight is even on both sitting bones and that your spine is lengthened in neutral.

Or: The Relaxation Position.

Action

1 Breathe in to prepare, and lengthen through your spine.

2 Breathe out as you squeeze your back passage (anus), as if trying to prevent yourself from passing wind, then bring this feeling forwards towards your pubic bone, as if trying to stop yourself passing urine. Ladies, you should be squeezing your vagina as well; gentlemen, you should feel your bladder being pulled upwards and your testicles may lift.

3 Breathe in and relax.

4 Wait for 4–5 seconds before trying again.

Repeat 10 times.

■ Try to keep your buttocks and leg muscles relaxed.

■ Also try to keep your jaw relaxed.

■ If you find the muscles tiring, stop and try again later.

Slow Zips (slow twitch)

Work up to being able to do 10 slow repetitions of the Wind Zip, holding for 10 seconds (women) and 5 seconds (men) each time before relaxing. With this Slow Zip, breathe normally throughout and do not hold your breath. Wait 4–5 seconds between zips.

Quick Zips (fast twitch)

Practise 10 quick repetitions of the Wind Zip. This time tighten and squeeze quickly as possible before releasing. Again, wait 4–5 seconds between zips. Breathe normally.

How often?

If you know that you have a pelvic-floor muscle problem, you should aim to do these exercises daily. You should notice an improvement after three to five months. If you do not, please visit your doctor, who can refer you to a women's health physiotherapist (they also work with men). Also, ladies, if you notice any increase in bulging in the vagina while doing the exercises, stop and consult your doctor.

To remind yourself to do your exercises, make them part and parcel of your day. Do them while you are waiting for the kettle to boil, in the ad breaks or even while waiting for a bus.

It is best to empty your bladder before trying these exercises.

Ladies

You are working up to doing 10 Slow Zips held for 10 seconds each time, followed by 10 Quick Zips, three times a day.

Gentlemen

You are working up to doing 10 Slow Zips held for 5 seconds, followed by 10 Quick Zips, three times a day.

RELEASING THE PELVIC FLOOR

It is possible for the pelvic floor to be overactive and tight, rather than underactive – for example, if you habitually sit with your legs crossed, or if, when practising Pilates, you turn your dimmer switch on full when it is not required.

Tension in the pelvic floor can compress the bladder, causing discomfort and urgency. It is important that you learn not only how to work the pelvic-floor muscles but also how to release them. Each time you practise these exercises, make sure that you fully relax the muscles between repetitions.

There are techniques you can use to help you release your pelvic floor. If you think these may be appropriate for you, mention this to your doctor. In the meantime, try this:

Pelvic-floor Release Exercise

Here you use deep abdominal breathing to help you relax your pelvic floor. The focus is very much on the in-breath.

Starting Position

Either sitting tall with your back supported or in the Relaxation Position; place your hands on your lower abdomen.

Action

1 Become aware of the ebb and flow of your breathing.

2 Breathe in through your nose and out through your mouth.

3 After each out-breath, take a moment's pause before you breathe in again.

4 Allow each out-breath to lengthen until it becomes twice as long as your in-breath.

5 Notice how your abdomen expands as you breathe in.

6 Allow your abdomen to expand fully as you breathe in. Allow your pelvic floor to release fully as you breathe in, and stay released as you breathe out.

- An empty bladder is essential.
- Do not try too hard... let go.
- Allow your sitting bones to open and widen.

PILES FOR MENTAL HEALTH

We have already discussed the impact of the mind on the body and the body on the mind. Through the regular practice of the Pilates for Life programme, we are hoping to help you achieve the perfect balance of mind and body.

STRESS

It is not stress itself which harms us (in fact, a degree of stress is integral to life itself), but our response to it, or rather how our bodies return to normal following a difficult situation. The body's 'fight-or-flight' response kicks in when we are faced with stressful situations – chemicals are produced to sharpen reactions and heighten the senses which, while essential to our survival in times of danger, can have a harmful effect if they remain in our bodies for too long.

Modern-day stresses come in different forms. They may be external factors such as illness, trauma, loss of a job or a loved one or money worries. And sometimes daily hassles mount up and you feel overloaded and unable to cope. Then there are the thoughts and feelings that can crop up, making you feel uneasy, inadequate and anxious or apprehensive. You may find your sleep patterns are disturbed, eating habits may be altered, you may eat too much or too little, you might grind your teeth or bite your nails or find release in drugs or alcohol. Physical symptoms can include increased heart rate, headaches, nausea, vomiting, indigestion, dry mouth, sweaty palms, a change in your breathing patterns and muscle tension, to list just a few!

When these feelings become so overwhelming that you no longer feel you can cope, there are lots of things that your doctor can recommend, including cognitive behavioural therapy, counselling, hypnotherapy and medication. Relaxation and breathing techniques have been shown to be very useful. And physical activity is hugely beneficial too – exercise burns up the adrenalin resulting from stress and frustration, and your body produces endorphins, which can promote feelings of happiness, while the chemical changes in the brain can help bring a greater sense of self-esteem, self-control, self-efficacy and confidence.

'The acquirement and enjoyment of physical wellbeing, mental calm and spiritual peace are priceless.'

Return to Life Through Contrology, **Joseph Pilates**

Pilates, with its principles of Concentration, Relaxation and Breathing, can be enormously beneficial in helping you cope with stress. The slow pace of the exercises offers a welcome contrast to the often hectic nature of our daily lives. By focusing on your breathing, you are encouraged to slow down and relax.

DEMENTIA AND ALZHEIMER'S

As we age, we have an increased risk of conditions such as dementia and Alzheimer's. Dementia is the name given to a group of related symptoms associated with an ongoing decline of the brain and its abilities, including:

- memory
- thinking
- language
- understanding
- judgement.

Usually dementia occurs in people who are 65 or over. The older you get, the more likely you are to develop it, and women are slightly more prone.

There are different types of dementia with different causes. The most common cause is Alzheimer's disease, but it can also be the result of a stroke or mini-stroke.

Dementia is progressive condition and there is currently no cure, although treatments can slow its progression.

Symptoms to look out for include:
■ remembering past events much more easily than recent ones
■ problems with thinking or reasoning, or finding it hard to follow conversations or TV programmes
■ feeling anxious, depressed or angry about memory loss, or feeling confused, even when in a familiar environment.

If you are worried about yourself, a friend or family member, you or they should speak to a doctor for a proper diagnosis as it can be difficult to distinguish these conditions from the normal memory loss associated with getting older.

Sufferers of dementia can benefit enormously from physical activity, and their physical health should not be ignored. For example, exercise can reduce the risk of falls in people with dementia and Alzheimer's, help to keep them mobile and can even be useful with later stages of dementia, although you may need to keep exercises simple. Remember also to encourage outdoor activities such as walking (accompanied).

DEPRESSION AND ANXIETY

Depression affects three times as many older people as dementia. It may be mild or severe and is often a side effect of an illness, loss of a loved one or a change in circumstances. Sometimes a well-deserved retirement can also spark a bout of depression, especially if a person misses their normal work routine. They may feel a lack of purpose.

Symptoms can be treated with cognitive therapy and medication, and exercise has an important role to play in some cases of depression. As we've seen, when you exercise you burn up the adrenalin produced by stress and frustration, and your body produces endorphins, which can promote feelings of happiness. Studies have shown that exercise can help people recover from depression and prevent them from becoming depressed in the first place.

EXERCISES TO BALANCE MIND AND BODY

Through enhanced awareness we hope to develop 'mindfulness', helping you become attuned to the way your mind and body feels both during the exercises and when going about your daily activities. Below are a few exercises chosen because they are particularly helpful in releasing mental tension and the physical tension it can lead to.

Recommended Exercises for Mental Health
■ Shoulder Drops (p. 46)
■ Chin Tucks and Neck Rolls (p. 26)
■ Nose Numbers (p. 164)
■ Spine Curls (p. 58)
■ Knee Rolls (p. 86)
■ Cat (p. 57)
■ Rest Position (p. 62)
■ Bow and Arrow (p. 67)
■ Side Reach with Breathing (p. 72)
■ Roll-downs Against a Wall (p. 104)
■ Breathing Exercises (pp. 168–69)
■ Thoracic Stretch Against the Wall (p. 170)
■ Standing Thoracic Rotation at the Wall (p. 171)

Guided Relaxation

This is a systematic relaxation exercise. Try to get someone with a calm, deep, gentle voice to read the cues for you or record them yourself.

Starting Position

You need to be in a comfortable position – you could be lying on your back, in which case have plenty of pillows supporting you (you might like one under your knees), or you could be side-lying or even sitting, as long as you are supported.

Action

Take your awareness down to your feet and soften the soles, uncurling the toes.

Soften your ankles.

Soften your calves.

Release your knees.

Release your thighs.

Allow your hips to open.

Allow the small of your back to open and release.

Feel and enjoy the length of your spine, but let it go.

Take your awareness down to your hands, stretch your fingers away from your palms, feel the centre of your palms opening.

Then allow your fingers to curl and your palms to soften.

Allow your elbows to open.

Allow the front of your shoulders to soften.

With each out-breath, allow your shoulder blades to widen.

Allow your breastbone to soften.

Allow your neck to release.

Check your jaw – it should be loose and free.

Allow your tongue to widen at its base and rest comfortably at the bottom of your mouth.

Your lips are softly closed.

Your eyes are softly closed.

Enjoy the soft darkness.

Your forehead is wide and smooth and free of lines.

Your face feels soft.

Your body feels soft and warm.

Allow your body to sink into the pillows supporting you.

Observe your breathing, but do not interrupt it – just enjoy its natural rhythm …

To come out of the relaxation: bring your awareness back to your breathing and observe its ebb and flow. Wriggle your fingers, then your toes. Take your time to move slowly (on to your side, if you are lying on your back). Do not rush back up to standing.

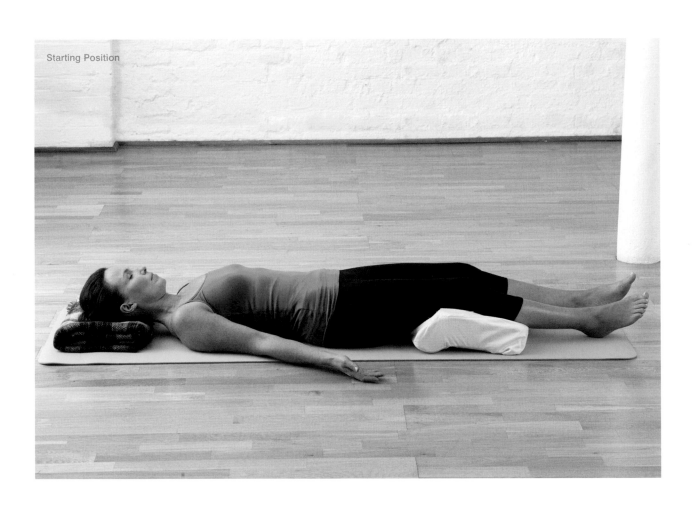

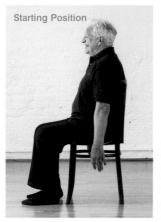 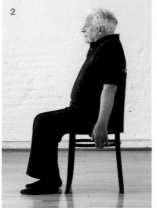 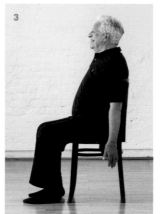 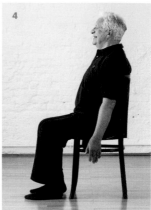

Shoulder Boxes

This is a great exercise to help you find the best position for your shoulders: one that is free from tension.

✱ Caution: take advice if you have neck or shoulder problems. ✱

Starting Position

Sit or stand tall with your arms by your sides.

Imagine a box positioned in front of your shoulders. We are going to trace the outline of the box with your shoulder tips.

Use an appropriate level of core connection to control your alignment and movements.

Action

1 Breathe in as you slide both shoulders forwards along the imagined bottom of the box.

2 Breathe out as you slide your shoulders up along the front edge of the box.

3 Breathe in as you slide your shoulders back along the top of the box.

4 Breathe out as you slide your shoulders down the back of the box.

Repeat 5 times.

■ Throughout the exercise stay lengthened in the spine.

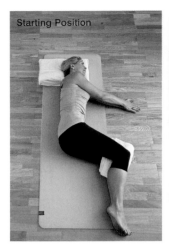 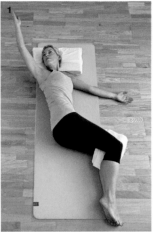 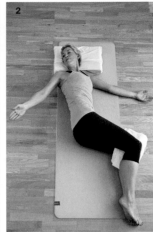 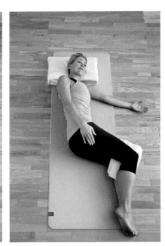

Chalk Circles

Probably the number-one feel-good exercise of the book, this mobilises the head, neck, torso and shoulders, opening you out across your upper body.

∗ Caution: take advice if you have back or shoulder problems. ∗

Starting Position

Side-lying on your left side, place a cushion/folded towel underneath your head to ensure that your head and neck are in line with your spine. Bend both knees in front of you, so that your hips and knees are bent to a right angle. (You may also place another cushion between your knees if you wish.) Lengthen both arms out in front of you at shoulder height, left arm resting on the mat and right arm on top of the left.

Use an appropriate level of core connection to control your alignment and movements.

Action

1 Breathe in and, keeping your right arm straight, begin to circle it in an arc above your head.

2 Breathe out as you continue to fully circle your arm around, allowing your head and neck and upper spine to rotate with the movement. Complete the circle of the arm and return your arm and spine back to the Starting Position.

Repeat up to 5 times, then repeat on the other side.

■ Note that it is unlikely that the hand of the circling arm will reach the floor (unless you are very flexible).

■ Check your side-lying starting position – shoulder above shoulder, hip above hip, knee above knee and foot above foot.

■ Ensure that your pelvis remains stable throughout.

■ Take care not to arch your back or tip your head back.

Rolling Chalk Circles

Clear the decks because in this fun version you get to roll around the floor, so you will need a lot of space. The aim is to achieve a fabulous stretch across your body. You are combining two exercises here: Hip Rolls (p. 66) and Chalk Circles (p. 183). We are less concerned with technique and more with freedom of movement and enjoyment.

If you find the breathing pattern difficult, just breathe normally.

✱ Caution: take advice if you have neck, back or shoulder problems. ✱

Starting Position

Relaxation Position, but with a substantial cushion under your head (a bed pillow is perfect), keeping your feet together and extending your arms to the sides.

Use an appropriate level of core connection to control your alignment and movements.

> ■ Enjoy the movements, but stay in control and take care not to overreach your arm or overarch your back.

Action

1 Breathe in and roll your knees across to the right. Simultaneously start to move your left hand across your hips to start the circle.

2 Breathe out as you roll on to your right side, knees still together; your left arm will continue its circle upwards.

3 Breathe in as you reach up and overhead.

4 Breathe out when you have to start rolling your body and knees back to the centre position; your arm continues its circle down and around to the Starting Position.

5 Breathe in as your knees roll left, your right arm starting to circle over your hip.

6 Breathe out as you roll on to your left side, knees still together; your right arm will continue its circle.

7 Breathe in as you reach up and overhead.

8 Breathe out when you have to start rolling back to the centre position; your right arm continues its circle down and around to the Starting Position.

Repeat as many times as you like!

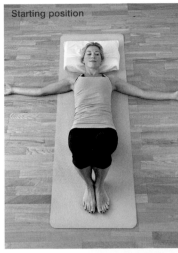

Starting position

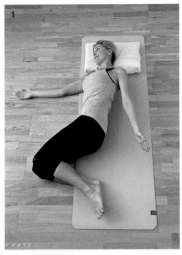

1

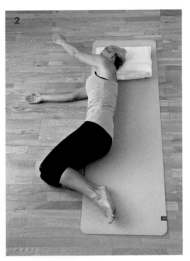

2

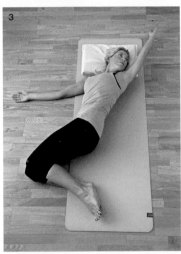

3

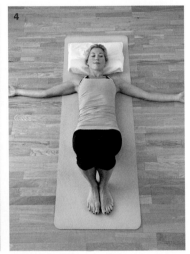

4

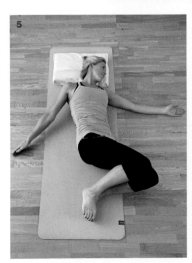

5

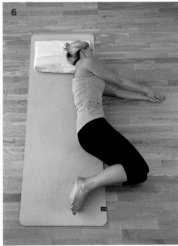

6

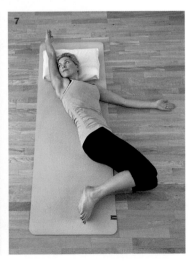

7

EXERCISING AFTER A STROKE

The medical term for a stroke is a cardiovascular accident – literally, an accident involving the blood supply to the brain. The brain needs a plentiful and constant supply of oxygen brought via the bloodstream in order to function well. In certain circumstances this can be interrupted, either by a clot stopping the immediate flow of blood to a given area of the brain, or by a rupture in a blood vessel within the brain, causing a bleed. The resultant damage depends on the severity of the blockage or bleed, and the function of the brain tissue that is damaged.

According to statistics, there are approximately 150,000 stroke victims each year in the UK; most sufferers are over the age of 50, although much younger people can be affected.

'Do something every day that is loving towards your body and allows you to enjoy the sensations of your body.'

Golda Poretsky

CAUSES AND CONSEQUENCES OF A STROKE

The commonest factors linked to having a stroke are high blood pressure, high cholesterol levels, obesity, smoking, diabetes, narrowing of arteries, lack of exercise, age and certain genetic factors.

In the main, the consequences of a stroke include:
■ facial weakness
■ muscle weakness affecting the voluntary movement, co-ordination and strength of the limb(s) on one side or complete paralysis of the arm and/or leg on one side
■ difficulty swallowing and speaking
■ difficulty making decisions
■ difficulty judging distances
■ poor body awareness
■ altered or complete loss of sensation in the arm and/or leg
■ memory changes
■ associated depression
■ possible changes in personality.

This list does not make for happy reading, but there is much that can be done for people who have suffered a stroke, so please read on!

✳ Recommended Exercises after a Stroke

In addition to the exercises on the following pages, those listed below may also be useful (with medical permission). Use your non-affected side to help if necessary:

■ Ribcage Closure (p. 47) – hold the affected side with the other hand and use it to lift the arm overhead
■ Starfish (p. 48) – hold the affected side with the other hand and use it to lift the arm overhead
■ Spine Curls (p. 58) or Bridge (p. 94) – to strengthen the hip
■ Shoulder Boxes (p. 182)
■ Leg Slides (p. 43)
■ Knee Openings (p. 43)
■ Single-knee Fold (p. 44)
■ Standing Balance (under supervision) (pp. 123–25)

RECOVERY AND PILATES
AFTER A STROKE

This depends on the severity of the stroke, but the general understanding is that recovery from a stroke can continue for up to two years after the incident. Many people do, however, continue to improve long after this time period, given strong motivation and the right sort of rehabilitation.

Pilates can be of great benefit to you if you are recovering from a stroke. You will need to be under the guidance of a medical practitioner who can give you individual encouragement and feedback. Many medical practitioners are also Pilates-trained.

After a stroke you may feel much less physically aware of one side of your body due to the changes in the brain, affecting your day-to-day movements. By continually being made aware of the whole body as you exercise (the correct alignment needed for each Pilates exercise will help to restore body awareness), your ability to control it may improve.

Pilates exercises can also encourage the proper working of groups of muscles around each joint, which can help with your co-ordination and the flow of movement. And of course, many Pilates exercises improve balance, which will help build confidence in walking and other daily activities. It is also important to include exercises which promote weight-bearing through the arm and leg as this will also stimulate the group action of muscles around the joints.

Progress may be slow, but it is worth persevering, as doing Pilates will also help improve and maintain your stamina through the day. You need to remember that everyone is different, and the effects of a stroke may vary greatly from one person to the next. Pilates can be tailored very easily to meet these individual needs, but always ask for medical clearance before starting any new form of exercise.

So to summarise, our primary goals here are to:
■ increase whole-body awareness through mindful, purposeful exercise, in particular correct static and dynamic alignment
■ encourage muscle control and precision of movement
■ improve balance and co-ordination
■ 'wake up' the affected side
■ encourage weight-bearing exercise.

As mentioned, these exercises should be done under the guidance of a medical practitioner until advised otherwise.

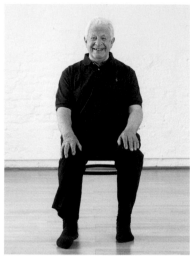

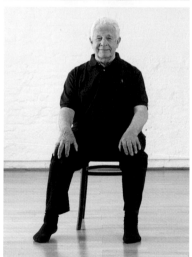

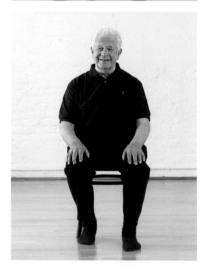

Foot Taps
This exercise helps to 'wake up' your affected side.

Starting Position
Sit tall on a sturdy chair (you will need to be fairly near the front) with your hands on your knees, feet hip-width apart and weight evenly balanced on both feet/sitting bones.

Use an appropriate level of core connection to control your alignment and movements.

Action
Breathe normally as you tap one foot in front of you, then out to the side and then behind. The speed and the distance the foot travels can be varied. Repeat 10 times in each direction, then repeat with the other leg.

Variation:
When you feel able to progress, you may try this exercise standing tall side-on to a wall for support (preferably with a rail or ledge to hold).

■ Maintain good posture; stay lengthened in the spine.

■ If you are seated, try to keep the weight even on both sitting bones.

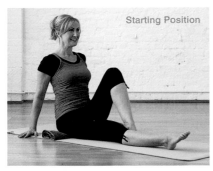
Starting Position

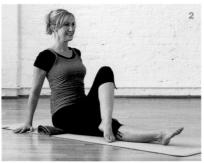
2

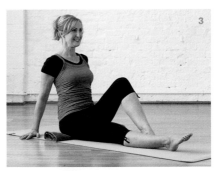
3

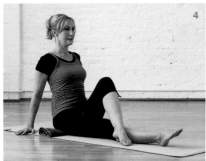
4

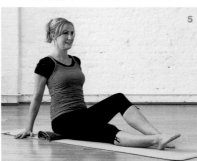
5

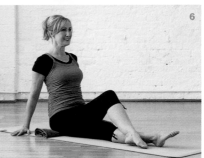
6

One Potato, Two Potato

This exercise, named for the old children's rhyme, helps you find the right placement for your affected foot. In the interest of balance, you should do it on both sides.

Starting Position

Either the Relaxation Position, or sit tall on your mat. You may sit on a rolled-up towel or cushion if it helps your alignment. You can also lean backwards slightly, resting on your hands, or lean your back against a wall. Have your right leg stretched out in front of you in line with your hip, your left leg bent in line with the hip.

Use an appropriate level of core connection to control your alignment and movements.

Action

Breathe normally as you tap the left foot either side of the right knee and continue tapping right and left as you slowly straighten the tapping leg out – tapping over the ankle, then working your way back up again.

Repeat 5 times, then repeat with the other leg.

■ Keep your weight even on both sitting bones as you tap away.

■ Maintain the length in your spine; do not collapse.

EXERCISING WITH PARKINSON'S

Parkinson's is a progressive neurodegenerative disease. In the UK, one in 500 people has the condition, and it is slightly more prevalent in men. Parkinson's is age-related, and is often diagnosed in people in their 70s. However, onset at a younger age, below the age of 40, can occur. It is caused by the loss of 80 per cent of brain cells that produce dopamine, a chemical messenger that carries signals into the brain. This lack of dopamine affects ability to control movement.

The characteristic signs of Parkinson's are bradykinesia, (slowness of movement), rigidity in muscles, a tremor (present at rest, decreasing with movement) and postural instability, which can lead to falls. There may be changes in posture, speech, handwriting and ability to move the facial muscles, as well as a lack of co-ordination. Gait is affected and there is a tendency to shuffle while walking. The brain struggles with the planning and execution of everyday motor performance. Although Parkinson's is considered as a movement disorder, it can also contribute to the development of non-motor disorders affecting the behaviour, cognition, emotion and autonomic and sensory system. The medications available improve the symptoms only. The variability and progression of the disease affect people differently, even in a single day.

Pilates empowers us to take control of the disease with a proactive approach. Typically, someone with Parkinson's will lose postural stability, balance and mobility. They may become round-shouldered with an increased curvature of the thoracic spine (kyphosis) and/or laterally flexed in standing position (Pisa syndrome) with a decrease of trunk rotation. We will be looking at correcting these problems. Prone-lying back extension and hip-extension exercises such as the Dart and Full Star are useful here (pp. 108 and 109), as are shoulder-opening exercises such as Windows and Bow and Arrow (pp. 91 and 67).

It must be kept in mind that if you have Parkinson's, you may struggle to balance and co-ordinate due to the postural shift and motor fluctuations. This is commonly known as 'on/off' syndrome and can best be described as an unpredictable shift from relative ease of movement (on) to a full stop (off).

It can also occur the other way round, moving suddenly to on.

On/off fluctuations are different from the phenomenon known as 'freezing' which can also affect people who have had Parkinson's for some time. 'Freezing' is the experience of stopping suddenly while walking or when beginning to initiate walking, and being unable to move forwards again for several seconds or minutes. People describe feeling as though their feet are 'frozen' or stuck to the ground, while the top half of their body still wants to move on. While freezing episodes tend to last for a short time, 'on/off' fluctuations can continue for minutes, or even hours. A person may have an air of general stillness with a reduction of body and hand gestures. Head and neck movements may also be restricted and initiating movement can be difficult, becoming increasingly slow and clumsy.

Parkinson's sufferers' ability to express personality or a sense of humour may be affected by the loss of verbal and non-verbal skills, and some may also experience slowing down of thinking, in much the same way as they might experience slowing down of movement. There may also be problems with the eyes, including blurred vision, double vision, excessive watering and dryness.

The gold-standard treatment for Parkinson's is pharmacological. However, exercise has been shown to be very successful in improving quality of life.
Our primary goals here are:

■ improve the motor skills needed for everyday living
■ improve the postural changes associated with Parkinson's
■ improve balance
■ improve co-ordination with rhythmic activities
■ increase flexibility
■ enhance breathing
■ encourage joint mobility, especially of the shoulders
■ improve ability to move from one position to the next
■ improve ability to safely turn
■ improve facial muscles
■ relax your muscle tone with supported positions (such as Relaxation Position and Side-lying).

Caution: Please consult with your medical practitioner before trying the exercises. Work safely, always position yourself near a wall or sturdy chair if standing and use cushions to support you in the other positions, as needed. Start with the exercises you find easiest in the most supported positions – probably Relaxation Position or Side-lying – progressing to seated and standing starting positions when you feel ready. Above all, enjoy the movements.

You may wear light, flexible, supportive shoes if you wish.

Recommended Exercises for Parkinson's

In addition to the exercises on the following pages, those listed below may also be useful (with medical permission).

- All Fundamental Exercises (pp. 20–83)
- Arm Swings (p. 104)
- Wall Push-ups (p. 102)
- Sliding Down the Wall (p. 100)
- Knee Rolls (p. 86)
- Crawling (p. 122)
- Lunge (p. 96)
- Functional Reaching (p. 130)
- Visual Skill Exercises (p. 78–81)
- Breathing Exercises (pp. 36–37)
- Weight Transfer Exercises (p. 126–29)
- Standing Balance (p. 123–5)
- Tipping Point (p. 129)
- Back Scratch and Neck Scratch (p. 140)
- Step Up (p. 208)
- Hands Exercises (p. 158–9)
- Full Star (p. 109)
- Lizard (p. 110)
- Bridge (p. 94)
- Windows (p. 91)
- Ankle Circles (p. 135)
- Eversion/Inversion (p. 134)
- Knee Opening with Band (p. 210)
- Seated Pillow Squeeze (p. 90)

Glue the Feet

For this exercise you have to imagine that your feet have been glued to the floor.

Starting Position

Stand tall with feet hip-width apart and arms by your sides. Have a chair alongside you in case you need it.

Use an appropriate level of core connection to control your alignment and movements.

Action

1 Breathe in as you force/press both feet into the floor.

2 Breathe out as you lift the right foot with force, imagining it has been fixed by glue to the floor.

3 Return your foot to the starting position.

Repeat, alternating right and left feet.

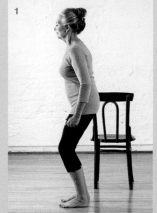 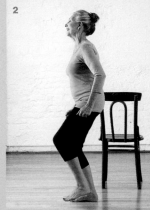

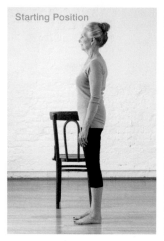

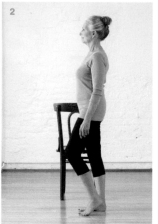

2

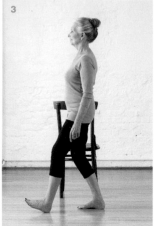

3

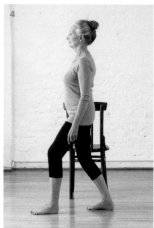

4

Stepping

The aim here is to control the way you step. It will help you to overcome problems you may experience of a quickening in your steps as you are walking, or if you have difficulty in initiating your steps. Read through the directions several times before attempting. You might find it more helpful to ask a friend to read you the directions or record them.

Starting Position

Stand tall. Check that your feet are hip-width apart and, if possible, parallel, that your legs are straight, but not locked and your pelvis and spine are in neutral. You may want to have a sturdy chair beside you.

Use an appropriate level of core connection to control your alignment and movements.

'You may have
Parkinson's disease,
but it does not
have you.'

Action

Breathe naturally throughout.

1 Move the weight of your body on to the right leg.

2 Bend your left leg at the knee and hip, so that you come up on to your left toes.

3 When the weight is fully on the right leg and your left one feels light, lift it off the floor and slowly step it forwards. As it is swinging forwards, pull your toes up, so that your heel lands on the ground first.

4 Slowly lower your toes down and gently allow your weight to transfer forwards on to the whole of the foot, with your left knee bending slightly as you do so. Do not let the right heel come off the ground and try not to let your body lean forwards at the hip.

5 Slowly return the weight back over the right foot until there is no weight on the left foot and it feels light and free enough to lift back to the Starting Position.

6 Swap legs and repeat 12 times.

Strategies for helping you cope with 'Freezing'

You may feel at times as though your feet are 'frozen', but that the top half of your body wants to keep going. This exercise will help train you to overcome these moments. You will need a rotating chair (like a standard office chair) for this exercise.

Starting Position

Sitting tall on the rotating chair, place your feet hip width-apart, arms comfortably on the armrests and look straight ahead. If your chair has no arm rests, fold your arms in front of you as for Waist Twists (p. 64).

Use an appropriate level of core connection to control your alignment and movements.

Action

Breathe naturally throughout the exercise.

1 Flex your feet as fast as possible without lifting the heels from the floor. Encourage the movement by calling 'Toes up – Foot go'. The response should be a sudden upward movement. Repeat 5 times.

2 Now add in rotating the chair slowly towards the right, back to centre and then left, allowing your feet to follow the movement. Repeat 6 times.

3 Then stand up and walk for 4 steps.

Variations

■ Make the chair rotate faster as you grow in confidence.
■ Standing against a wall, lift the toes, alternating right and left; then alternate heel and toes. Move away from the wall and, maintaining the movement of the feet, rotate your trunk as quickly as you can, letting the pelvis accomplish the movement.

> ■ Keep the upright position throughout the movements, neither swaying backwards nor slumping forwards.
>
> ■ Keep your weight centred and balanced evenly on both sitting bones, allowing your head to balance on top of your spine, looking straight ahead.

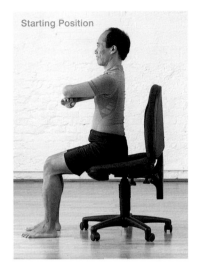
Starting Position

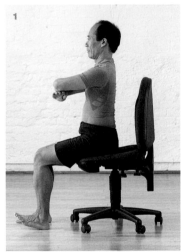
1

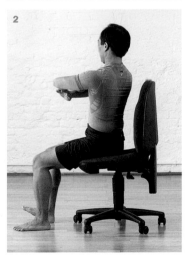
2

Step and Stop

This exercise will help with your initiation of movement, as well as with freezing.

Starting Position

Stand tall with one foot forwards, your arms in an opposite-arm swing position, e.g. right leg forwards, left arm forwards.

Use an appropriate level of core connection to control your alignment and movements.

Action

Breathe naturally.

1 Walk forwards for 6 steps, then stop.

2 Hold the position for 10 seconds, then start walking for another 6 steps.

Repeat the above 5 times.

Variations

■ Increase or decrease the number of steps, and increase the time you hold the position.
■ If you feel confident with the movement, repeat the sequence in a circle and increase the step length.
■ Play rhythmical music in the background to add more precision to your step/stop action.

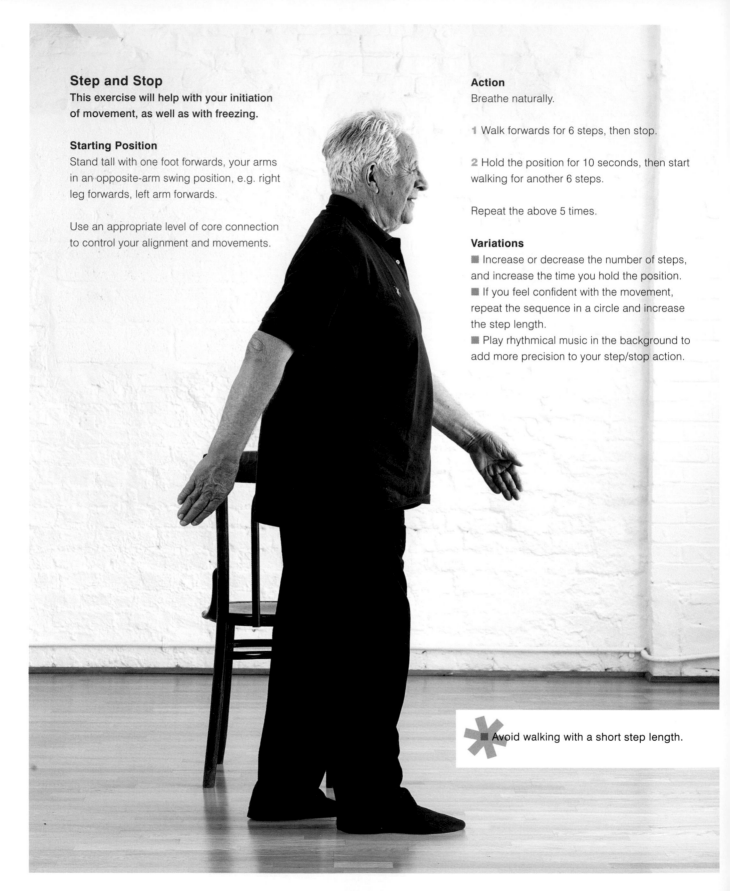

■ Avoid walking with a short step length.

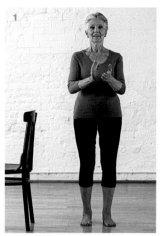
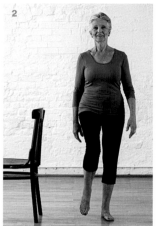
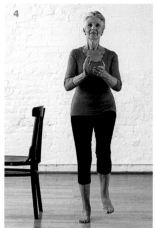
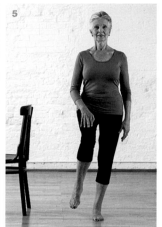

Walking and Clapping the Leg

The aim of this exercise is help you to overcome 'freezing' while walking, seated or turning. It requires you to clap your hands to a rhythm, so it helps to choose a favourite song with a steady beat.

Starting position

Stand tall on the floor. You may have a chair alongside you if you wish. Check that your pelvis and spine are in neutral, your feet are parallel, hip-width apart and your legs are straight.

Use an appropriate level of core connection to control your alignment and movements.

Action

Breathe normally throughout.

1 Start to clap your hands to a steady rhythm.

2 Stop the clapping and start marching on the spot. Try to match your marching to the rhythm of your clapping.

3 When you are ready and confident with the marching, add the clapping to your marching.

4 Clap and march with the same rhythmical tempo.

5 Once you have found the pattern, start to walk, clapping the leg you would like to step forwards or backwards.

6 Walk forwards, alternating right and left feet for 10 steps.

7 Now try walking backwards as above.

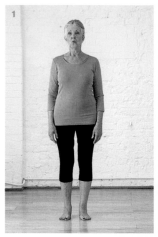
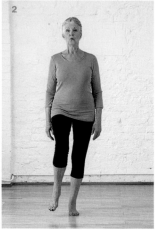
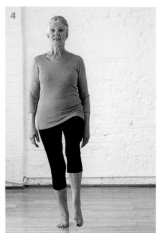
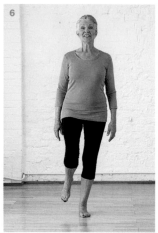

Walking and Talking

It might sound strange to have to practise this, but it really is effective.

Starting Position

Standing tall, check that your pelvis and spine are in neutral, your feet are parallel, hip-width apart, and your legs are straight. Your arms should be by your sides.

Use an appropriate level of core connection to control your alignment and movements.

Action

Breathe normally throughout.

1 Start to call out numbers to a steady rhythm and with a loud and clear voice.

2 Start marching on the spot. Try to match your marching to the rhythm of your voice.

3 When you are confident with the marching, count your steps out loud and march with the same rhythmical tempo.

4 Once you have found the pattern, start to walk forwards.

5 Walk forwards, alternating starting on right and left feet for 10 steps.

6 Now try to count backwards as you repeat Action 5, walking backwards.

7 You are now ready to count backwards while walking forwards and vice versa.

Variations

■ You may use a metronome to keep the rhythm and make the walking faster or slower.
■ Choose your favourite song and sing it loudly, to improve your breathing pattern too.
■ Keep swinging your arms throughout.

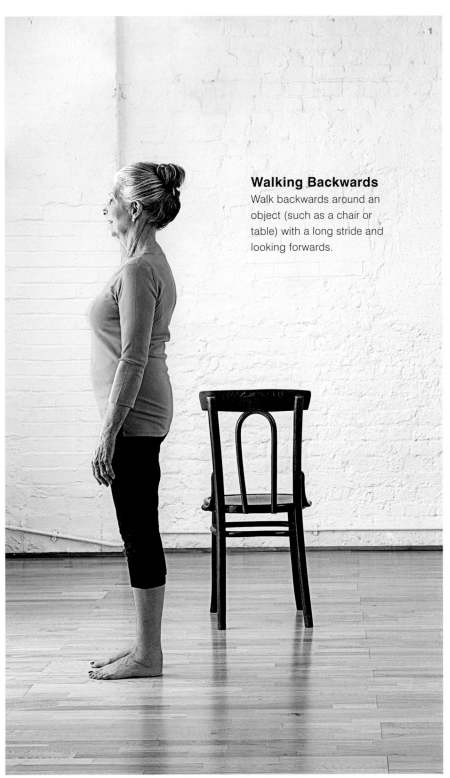

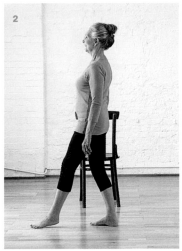

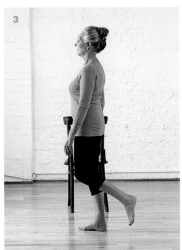

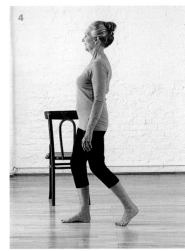

Walking Backwards

Walk backwards around an object (such as a chair or table) with a long stride and looking forwards.

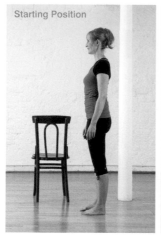 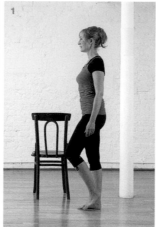 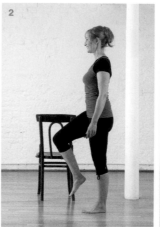 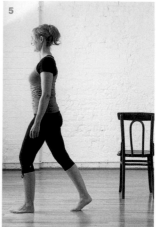

Strategy for Crossing Obstacles

Starting Position
Standing tall, check that your pelvis and spine are in neutral, your feet are parallel, hip-width apart and your legs are straight. Your arms should be by your sides.

Action
Breathe normally throughout.

1 Start to walk on the spot to a steady rhythm.

2 Try to walk and lift one foot higher every fourth step.

3 When you are ready and confident with the walking and the lifting, walk moving forwards.

4 Walk and lift the foot higher.

5 Once you have found the pattern, start to place the lifted foot with a longer step. Your step length will increase, but always stay balanced.

6 Walk forwards, alternating right and left feet for 10 steps.

7 Now try walking backwards, as above.

8 Now try walking on a diagonal.

Variation: Hold a walking stick upside down (with its handle on the floor) and step over the handle. Your brain will process the obstacle and its response will be to lift the foot. Place the stick's handle on a sticky mat to prevent it from sliding.

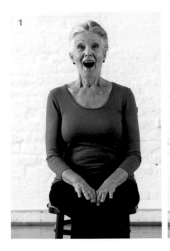
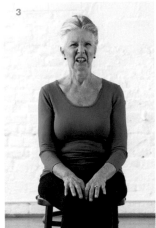
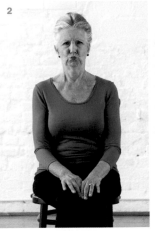
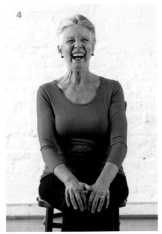

Facial Exercises

These might not be the most glamorous exercises in the book, but they are important, as they help to keep your face mobile. They will also help to improve your facial muscles and thus help you get your smile back.

Starting Position

Sit on a sturdy chair or stand tall. If seated, place your hands on your thighs and lengthen up through the crown of the head. Look straight ahead as though into a mirror.

Action

Pull the following faces:

1 Surprise – lift your eyebrows and open your mouth.

2 Displeasure – frown and purse your lips together.

3 Disgust – crinkle your nose as if you're smelling something truly awful.

4 Pleasure – smile as broadly as you can.

Variation: Try these exercises with a friend and then add a laugh; it helps with the breathing, too. First one to laugh buys the drinks (OK, organic tea).

Variation
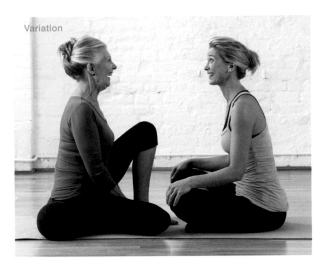

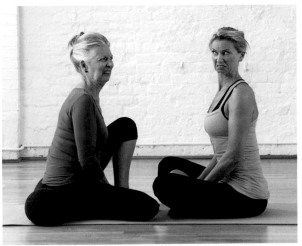

MULTIPLE SCLEROSIS

Multiple Sclerosis (MS) is most commonly diagnosed in people aged 25–35, but we have included it in this book as it can occur at any age and it causes long-term disability, for which some Pilates exercises may be useful.

MS is an autoimmune disease, which means the immune system attacks other cells within the body. In MS the insulating cells of the nerves are attacked, leading to changes in the ability to move. It affects approximately 100,000 people in the UK.

Our central nervous system is made up of the brain and the spinal cord. Nerves exit from the spinal cord at every vertebral level to go to every part of our bodies, taking electrical impulses to our muscles and bringing back information, which is then processed in the brain. Nerve fibres are completely covered with a sort of insulating material known as myelin. The myelin is arranged around the nerves in a certain way that not only protects the nerve but which also speeds up the passage of the electrical impulse along the nerve.

In MS, the immune system attacks the myelin and damages it, and strips it off the nerve fibres, leaving scars along the nerve known as lesions or plaques. This has the effect of disrupting the passage of the impulses either partially or completely. The nerve fibres may also be damaged, leading to increased disability over time. The symptoms can vary from person to person, but the main ones are progressive difficulty in moving, altered sensation, changes to speech and swallowing, balance problems, dizziness and fatigue. MS is also characterised by relapses and remissions.

BENEFITS OF PILATES WITH MS

The aims of any exercise regime for anyone with MS include keeping a good range of movement, maintaining good strength and balance, helping co-ordination and maintaining an upright posture, to name but a few. Exercising may help to manage fatigue as well as improving mood. Pelvic floor exercises will be of great benefit to ensure good bladder control as we age.

Our primary goals are to:
- maintain the range of movement of your joints
- improve your muscle strength
- enhance your body awareness and co-ordination skills
- improve your balance
- improve your posture and postural stability
- increase your pelvic floor control
- improve your mood

Cautions
- If you are having a relapse it may not be advisable to carry on exercising until you have recovered so, as always, do take medical advice.
- If you are heat sensitive due to the MS, do ensure that the room you are exercising in is cool and well ventilated.
- Take short breaks during your exercise regime to prevent fatigue.
- Your symptoms and the side effects of medication may vary throughout the day, so consider this when deciding which time of day to exercise.

EXERCISES FOR MULTIPLE SCLEROSIS

Please seek medical permission to exercise. The following exercises may be included in your workouts.

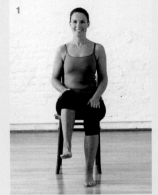
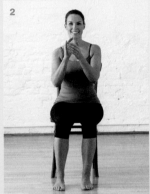

Recommended Exercises for MS

Which exercises you choose will depend largely on how you are feeling and may vary on a daily basis. Try to do a balanced workout. With medical permission you might like to try the exercises for Parkinson's (pp. 191–99) plus the following:

- Breathing exercises standing (p. 168–69)
- Pelvic-floor exercises (p. 176–77)
- Foot exercises (pp. 132–135)
- Foot Drag (p. 215)
- Leg Slides (p. 43)
- Seated C-curve (p. 56)
- Climb a Tree Preparation (p. 112)
- Knee Openings (p. 43)
- Spine Curls (p. 58)
- Bridge with Marching Feet (p. 95)
- Hip Rolls (p. 66)
- Cat (p. 57)
- Hip Hinge (p. 74)
- Table Top Preparation (p. 50)
- Full Table-top (p. 111)
- Zig-zags (p. 88)
- Seated Bow and Arrow (p. 68)
- Side-lying Leg Lift and Lower (p. 115), Bicycle (p. 117), Knee Cross-overs (p. 116)
- Dart (p. 108)
- Lizard (p. 110)
- Full Star (p. 109)
- Weight Transfer Exercises (pp. 126–29)
- Standing on One Leg (p. 53)
- Sliding Down the Wall (p. 100)
- Pilates Squat (p. 75)
- Lunge and its variations (p. 96)
- Hand Exercises (pp. 136–37)
- Side Reach (p. 70)

Stamping Ground and Clap

Starting Position
Sit or stand tall.

Use an appropriate level of core connection to control your alignment and movements.

Action
Breathe normally throughout.

1 Start to stamp your right foot and then the left, and repeat.

2 After each stamp add a clap: stamp-clap-stamp-clap-stamp-clap-stamp-clap.

3 Then stamp-clap-clap-stamp-clap-clap-stamp-stamp.

4 Then try clap-stamp-stamp-clap-stamp-clap-clap-stamp.

You can enjoy discovering all the possible combinations.

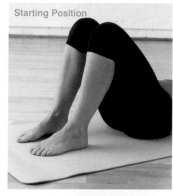

Starting Position

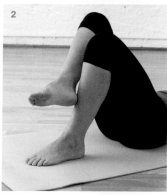

1

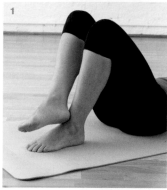

2

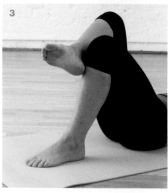

3

Shin Slide

To improve your proprioception and control.

Starting Position

Lie in the Relaxation Position with feet hip-width apart and parallel. Bring your awareness to the position of the feet.

Use an appropriate level of core connection to control your alignment and movements.

Action

Breathe normally throughout.

1 Reach with the right heel to the left ankle and return the right foot, precisely, to the same place in the Starting Position.

2 Repeat the above, but touch in the middle of the shin and return the foot back to the Starting position precisely.

3 Repeat the above, but touching higher on the shin, then return the foot to the Starting Position.

4 Once you have mastered the pattern precisely, slide the heel along the shin and return to the Starting Position.

Repeat 8 times with each leg.

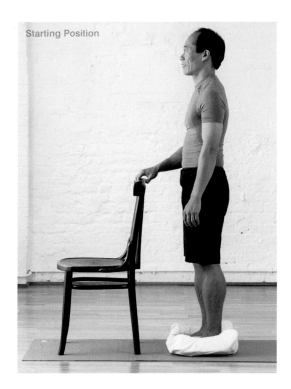

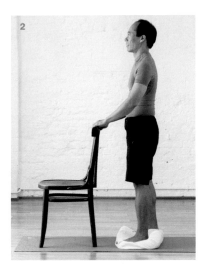

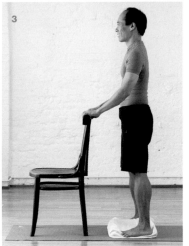

Pillow Balance
To improve your balance and proprioception.

Starting Position

Stand tall on a soft pillow with one hand on a sturdy chair.

Use an appropriate level of core connection to control your alignment and movements.

Action

Breathe normally throughout.

1 Balance on the pillow for 10 seconds with the eyes opened and then closed, holding the chair lightly but as needed.

2 Repeat the above with an off-set stance (one foot in front).

3 Repeat the above with a wide off-set stance.

4 Repeat the above in a one-leg standing position.

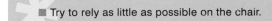

✳ ■ Try to rely as little as possible on the chair.

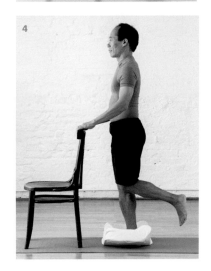

EXERCISING WITH AND AFTER BREAST CANCER

Breast cancer is now the most common female cancer in the Western world. Surgery is often the first line of attack, and additional treatment options may include radiotherapy, chemotherapy and hormonal treatments. These may take their toll both physically and emotionally, and commonly reported symptoms include fatigue (tiredness), loss of physical fitness, reduced arm mobility, anxiety and diminished self-confidence.

Historically, women have been told to rest while undergoing treatment and to avoid physical activity; but we now know that this message is unhelpful and that exercise and physical activity play an important role in the recovery and rehabilitation of women with breast cancer, helping with energy levels, strengthening muscles, mobilising stiff joints and improving self-confidence and body image.

Pilates is an excellent choice for women in the recovery phase from breast cancer due to its focus on education of movement and improving mobility and core stability. Pilates can be integrated into rehabilitation packages from about 12 weeks post-surgery, as long as there are no immediate concerns from the medical team.

For many women, the main goal of rehabilitation is to optimise their functional ability and return to all activities previously enjoyed; this may or may not involve return to work and sporting pastimes. The main focus is often on the upper body as surgery and radiotherapy can result in scarring and loss of mobility in the shoulder region. However, it is important not to neglect the rest of the body because cancer treatments can also result in general deconditioning. Pilates is an excellent discipline for tackling these challenges in a holistic way.

JOSEPH PILATES AND EVE GENTRY

In 1955 one of Joseph Pilates's first disciples, Eve Gentry, underwent a radical mastectomy and, as a professional dancer, she was frustrated by the resulting lack of mobility. Arriving at Joe's studio after the operation, she showed him how limited her shoulder movements were. His response? 'Don't worry. We fix.'

And 'fix' he did. There is fabulous archival footage of Eve moving through workouts, in which she is seen doing advanced exercises. However, when Joe submitted this for review by doctors at a hospital with which he wanted to make an alliance, the doctors came back to him saying that Eve's level of recovery was impossible. In response, Joe and Eve filmed more footage, in which she performed the routines shirtless. (Some of that footage can be seen on the archival film as well.) Eve was able to return to professional dancing and teaching.

✳ Recommended Exercises for Breast Health

The following exercises are particularly recommended, but please take medical advice.

- Relaxation Position (p. 23)
- Guided Relaxation (p. 180)
- Shoulder Drops (p. 46)
- Shoulder Boxes (p. 182)
- Chin Tucks & Neck Rolls (p. 26)
- Thumb Rolls (p. 77)
- Dumb Waiter with Medial Rotation (p. 105)
- Walking on the Wall Up and Down (p. 103)
- Ribcage Closure (p. 47)
- Floating Arms (p. 52)
- Arm Circles in Relaxation Position and Standing (p. 92)
- Waist Twist in Standing Position (p. 64)
- Seated Thoracic Extension (p. 153)

PILATES EXERCISES FOLLOWING BREAST-CANCER SURGERY

It is vital that you check with your medical practitioner before you start to exercise. As mentioned above, if you feel able, you could include some of the exercises below from about 12 weeks post-surgery with your doctor's permission.

Our primary goals are to:
- increase your ability to carry out normal activities
- improve your shoulder flexion (bringing the arm up in front of you)
- improve your shoulder abduction (taking the arm out to the side)
- improve your medial rotation (turning the arm inwards)
- strengthen your back muscles
- improve your trunk rotation
- stretch your anterior wall.

It is important, as always, to do the exercises within your pain-free range of movement, never pushing into pain. Be patient; your range of movement will improve with time.

EXERCISING WITH A HIP REPLACEMENT

Having a new hip is now a common and relatively trouble-free operation. Simply put, having a hip replacement means that the bony end of your femur or leg bone is removed and replaced with a metal one commonly known as a prosthesis. The bony part of the hip socket in the pelvis is also removed and replaced with a new socket.

Most people are offered a new hip because the pain and lack of mobility in their joint severely impacts their normal life. Often osteoarthritis (p. 158) is the reason for this pain but it can also be due to old injury, rheumatoid arthritis, gout, and obesity.

After the operation, pain is generally much reduced and mobility at the joint is restored, though there are a few movements which should still be avoided for a period of time after the operation as they have the potential to cause a dislocation of the new joint. These movements are listed below, but you should check with your consultant and/or physiotherapist before you start to exercise again, as recommendations may differ from surgeon to surgeon and according to which type of surgery you have had.

Movements to avoid may include:

■ rotating the hip fully outwards (that is, turning your leg out completely on your operated side)
■ bringing your leg across the midline of your body
■ full hip flexion to the chest (that is, bringing the leg up past 90 degrees)
■ turning your thigh bone inwards at the hip (internal rotation)
■ the combined movements of hip flexion, adduction (bringing the leg in towards the midline) and internal rotation.

EXERCISING WITH A NEW HIP

The most important thing is to work on the muscles around the joint in order to strengthen them so that they support the new hip and restore normal movement.

Often particular muscles around the hip joint become weak because of the pain in the arthritic joint before you even had the operation. This affects the way you use the joint and can change the way you walk and move around. Chances are that you will have avoided putting too much weight on the affected side for some time, the other hip having taken the strain (and with it the knee, ankle and foot). After the operation, you will have been given a stick to help you move around which will also change your walking pattern.

Most commonly affected are the muscles at the side of the hip, and those at the back of the joint, namely the tensor fascia lata and the gluteal muscles. The main muscle of power at the hip which is used when we walk is the large gluteus maximus and this can become very wasted and weak without you realising it. If your buttock muscle becomes weaker, often due to a sedentary lifestyle or a job involving a lot of bending, you may notice tightness developing in the hamstrings (at the back of your thighs). The main job of the hamstring muscle is to bend your knee rather than extend the hip, hence the change in your walking pattern. It is really important to get the gluteal muscles strengthened again to restore a good walking pattern and to make sure you can squat down and get up again without difficulty.

So, remembering the movements we need to avoid after a hip replacement, our main focus will be on improving and maintaining the hip's range of movement through:

- flexion (bringing the knee in towards the body)
- abduction (taking the leg to the side)
- extension (taking the leg behind)
- building strength in the weakened muscles, especially the buttock muscles.

Caution: it is important, as always, to do the exercises within your pain-free range of movement, never pushing into pain. This will improve over time and with careful and safe movements; you may need to adapt some of the Starting Positions, so that they are safe and comfortable for you. Take care getting down to the mat and up. Use your own strategy, depending on your limitations.

EXERCISES FOR HIP HEALTH

Please check with your medical practitioner before exercising. With medical permission, the following exercises may be added to your workout.

Recommended Exercises for Hip Health

- Leg Slides (p. 43)
- Star Preparation (p. 49)
- Prone Knee Lift (p. 49)
- Oyster – place a pillow between your knees to prevent the leg coming across the midline (p. 51)
- Tennis Ball Rising (p. 76)
- Spine Curls (p. 58)
- Sliding Down the Wall (p. 100)
- Bridge (p. 94)
- Full Table-top (p. 111)
- Side-lying Legs Lift and Lower – place a cushion under your top leg to prevent it from lowering too far and crossing your midline (p. 115)
- Standing Star hip abduction and extension (p. 118)

'We don't stop playing because we grow old. We grow old because we stop playing.' **George Bernard Shaw**

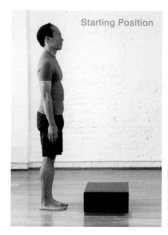 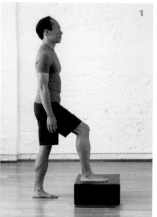 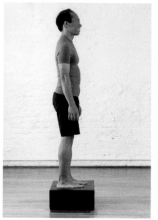 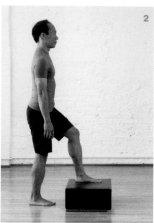

Step Up

This exercise will help improve your hip function. It will also increase your awareness of good hip, knee and ankle alignment. And it will help you climb the stairs.

Starting Position

Stand tall on the floor in front of a sturdy step or box, feet hip-width apart and parallel, arms by your sides. Have a sturdy chair beside you, if necessary.

Use an appropriate level of core connection to control your alignment and movements.

Action

Breathe normally throughout.

1 Lift the knee of the unaffected (unoperated) leg/hip and place the foot on the step followed by the affected leg.

2 Step back with the affected leg first, followed by the unaffected one.

(Remember this phrase as you climb the stairs: the good go up to heaven, the bad go down to hell.)

Progression: Step off the other side of the box with the affected leg followed by the unaffected one.

■ Avoid bending forwards with the spine or hinging backwards.

■ Keep the alignment of the head, spine and pelvis.

■ Avoid rolling the knees outwards or inwards.

■ Place the foot on the step and distribute the weight well before stepping up.

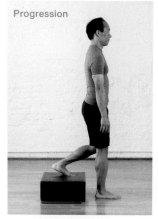 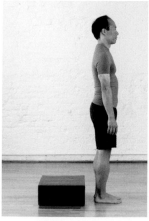

Progression

Big Squeeze

This exercise will mobilise your hips and activate your gluteals. You will need to be able to get down on to the floor or an exercise bench.

✳ Caution: if you have osteoporosis, you may wish to place a flat cushion under your abdomen. ✳

Starting Position

Lie prone with your legs straight and very slightly turned in from the hip. This means that, depending on the size of your feet, your big toes are touching. Place (or get a friend to place) a cushion between the tops of your thighs. Rest your forehead on your folded hands or on a flat cushion if it is more comfortable. Your upper body should stay open.

Use an appropriate level of core connection to control your alignment and movements.

Action

1 Breathe in to prepare to move.

2 Breathe out as you bring your legs together into parallel (squeezing the pillow between your thighs or simply feeling your inner thighs and gluteal muscles connecting).

3 Breathe in and release.

Repeat up to 10 times.

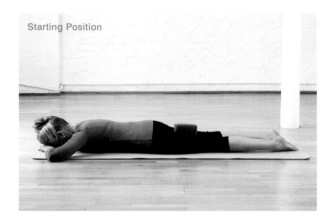

Starting Position

> ✳ ■ Your feet should stay on the ground.
>
> ■ Lengthen your legs as you squeeze, but do not lock out your knees.

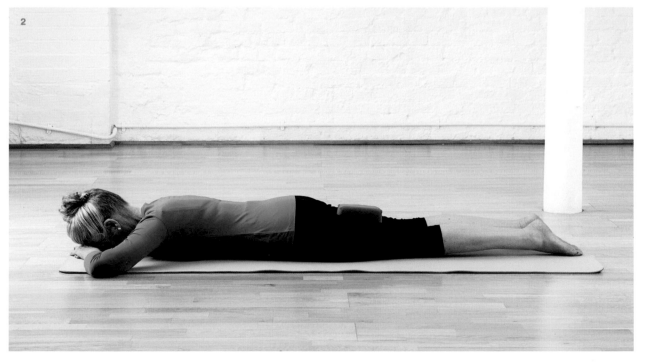

2

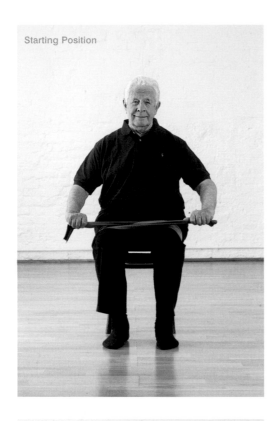

Starting Position

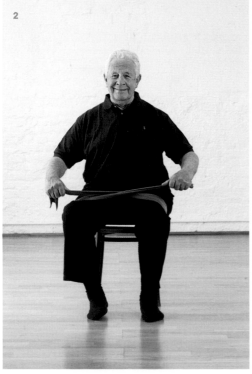

2

Seated Knee Openings with Band

As with Big Squeeze (p. 209), the aim is to mobilise the hip joints, while activating the gluteals. You will need to remember what you learned in Knee Openings (p. 43) and Oyster (p. 51). We will work both hips here. You will need a stretch band.

Starting Position

Sit tall on a sturdy chair, feet and knees hip-width apart and parallel (place your feet on a few books or a step if you are short in the leg). Place a stretch band around your thighs. Check that your weight is even on both sitting bones.

Use an appropriate level of core connection to control your alignment and movements.

Action

1 Breathe in to prepare to move.

2 Breathe out as you turn your thigh out from the hip in a knee-opening action. The action comes from the hip joint; you should feel your deep gluteals working.

3 Breathe in and return the leg to parallel with control.

4 Breathe out and turn out the other leg.

5 Breathe in and return the leg to the Starting Position with control.

Repeat up to 10 times

Variation: this exercise may also be done in the Relaxation Position, following the Actions above.

■ As you turn out the leg, ensure that you stay lengthened in the spine.

■ You must control the return action of the leg to avoid it springing back too far.

■ Your shoulders must stay open, collarbones wide, neck and jaw released.

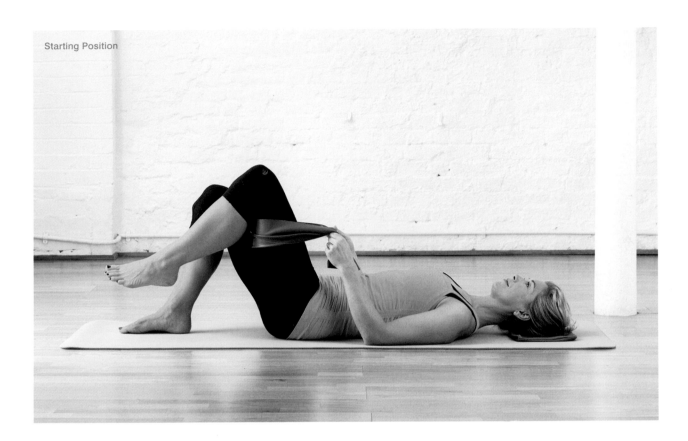

Knee Fold with Band/Scarf – Hip Extension
Our focus here is on improving hip extension. You will need a stretch band or scarf.

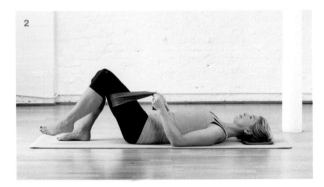

Starting Position
Relaxation Position. With control, fold one knee in (taking care not to pass 90 degrees) and wrap the band or scarf around your upper thigh. Hold with both hands, keeping your shoulders and collarbones wide and open.

Use an appropriate level of core connection to control your alignment and movements.

Action
1 Breathe in to prepare your body to move.

2 Breathe out as you press your leg away, resisting with the band/scarf.

3 Breathe in as you relax. Repeat 10 times with both legs.

- Keep your pelvis and spine still and centred throughout.
- Press away with the back of your thigh.
- Keep your leg directly in line with your hip joint.

EXERCISING WITH A KNEE REPLACEMENT

Having a knee replacement is becoming more common, with over 70,000 operations being performed each year in the UK. Reasons for having such a replacement are most often because of the pain and damage resulting from osteoarthritis (p. 156), but can also be due to gout, haemophilia, and rheumatoid arthritis (p. 157).

There are two types of knee replacement operations: a total replacement, or a partial replacement, where only one side of the knee joint is replaced. The knee joint is a complex joint and, because of this complexity, knee replacements are not as simple as total hip replacements. During the operation, the damaged bone on both the femur and the tibia is removed and replaced by a prosthetic metal surface. A spacer is also put in to mimic the action of the knee cartilage.

PILATES FOR KNEE REPLACEMENTS

The aims of the Pilates exercises here are to improve the strength of the thigh muscle, front and back, while increasing and maintaining a functional range of movement within the knee. Balance exercises will also be important, as you may have had a limp before the operation and we need to make sure the limp disappears!

EXERCISING AND RECOVERY

Your recovery should be under the care of your consultant who will tell you when you are ready to take up Pilates. This medical permission is essential. Each person is different, but most have full knee extension the day after surgery and 90-degree flexion by three days after surgery. You should be able to walk without a crutch or cane by 3 months post op.

Cautions:
■ Any exercises which entail kneeling will be uncomfortable and should be avoided.

■ Avoid squatting or lunging.
■ Spine Curls and Bridges may need to be avoided as they can put a strain on the tibia while the pelvis is lifting away from the floor.

Our exercise priorities are to:
■ restore full knee extension
■ restore knee flexion past 90 degrees
■ strengthen the quadriceps (front of thigh muscles)
■ improve your walking gait, by working on ankle and foot mobility as well as hip stability and mobility
■ correct any limping
■ improve your balance (when ready)
■ improve the rotation of your pelvis and thoracic spine.

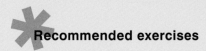

Recommended exercises

Please do not neglect the rest of your body! You will still be able to do many of the exercises in this book. For example the shoulder mobility and arm exercises. You may need to adjust the Starting Positions to be more comfortable. With medical permission, you may try the exercises on the following pages. **Moving on...**
When most of the swelling has subsided and the pain has lessened you can progress to the following exercises.

■ Very small (that is, within your available pain-free range) Pilates Squat (p. 75)
■ Very small Sliding Down the Wall (p. 100)
■ Small Mini (Partial) Lunge (p. 96)
■ Step Up (p. 208)

Foot Pedal

Starting Position

Sit tall or lie on your mat with both legs straight and hip-width apart.

Use an appropriate level of core connection to control your alignment and movements.

Action

Breathe normally throughout.

1 Point one foot and flex the other simultaneously.

2 Push the affected/operated knee gently down against the mat and hold the knee straight for 5 seconds, still breathing... then relax.

Repeat 5 times; less if you feel pain or discomfort.

Straight leg Raise
Before trying this, practise the exercises on p.214.

Starting Position

Choose one of the Starting positions above.

Use an appropriate level of core connection to control your alignment and movements.

Action

Breathe normally throughout.

1 With your affected knee straight, push it down in to the mat.

2 Pull your toes up towards you and slowly raise your straight leg about 20cm off the mat.

3 Hold for 5 seconds, still breathing, and lower.

Repeat 8 times.

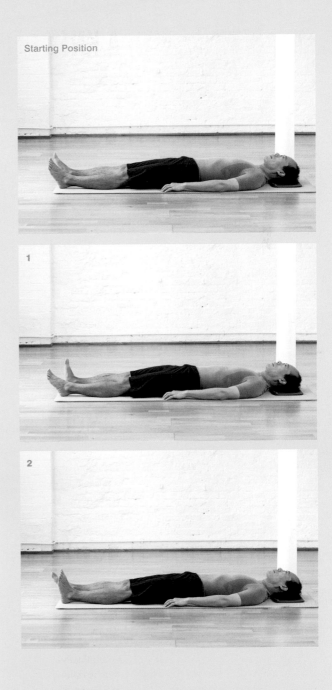

Starting Position

1

2

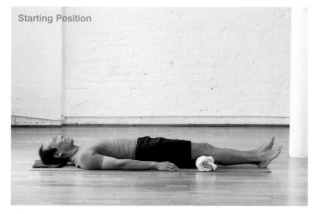

Starting Position

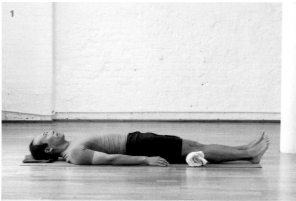

1

Towel under the knee

Starting position

Lie on your mat in the Relaxation position, feet hip-width apart, with your affected leg straight. Place a rolled-up towel under the affected knee. Your heel should rest on the mat.

Use an appropriate level of core connection to control your alignment and movements.

Action

Breathe normally throughout.

1 Push gently into the towel to straighten the affected knee, keeping the back of your knee on the towel and raising your heel off the mat.

2 Hold for 5 seconds, still breathing... then relax.

Repeat 8 times

Heel on the Towel

Starting position

Lie on your mat in the Relaxation position, legs hip-width apart but with your affected leg straight. Place a rolled-up towel under the heel of the affected leg. Allow your heel to rest on the towel.

Use an appropriate level of core connection to control your alignment and movements.

Action

Breathe normally throughout.

1 Push gently into the towel to straighten the affected knee.

2 Hold for 5 seconds, still breathing... and relax.

Repeat 8 times.

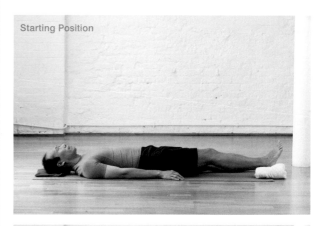

Starting Position

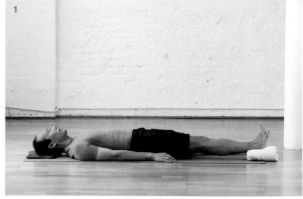

1

Foot Drag

Starting Position
The Relaxation Position, or sit tall on a chair, feet hip-width apart. Place a sliding cushion, or a plastic sheet, under the heel of your affected leg.

Use an appropriate level of core connection to control your alignment and movements.

Action
Breathe normally.

Bend your affected knee by sliding your foot forwards and backwards. Work within the range of movement that is available to you and is not painful.

Repeat 8 times.

Variation: If you find bending difficult, try putting a stretch band or scarf around your foot and, as you slide your foot, assist the movement by pulling on the band/scarf.

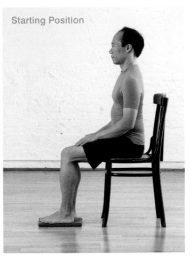

Starting Position

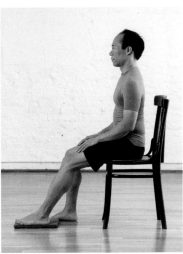

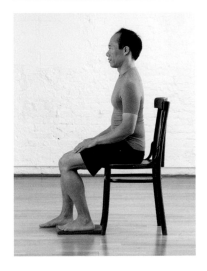

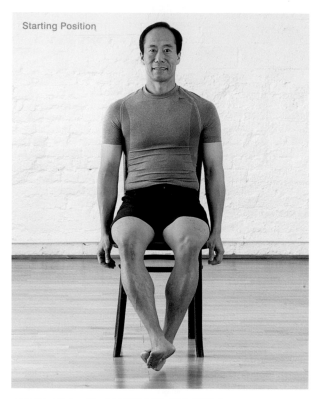

Starting Position

Supported Knee Flexion/Extension

Starting position

Sit tall on a sturdy chair. Your feet are away from the floor and your ankles crossed, with the ankle of the unaffected leg underneath.

Use an appropriate level of core connection to control your alignment and movements.

Action

Breathe normally throughout.

1 Start to straighten both knees. The unaffected leg will facilitate the movement and act as a support for the affected knee, pushing it gently.

2 As you return the legs towards the starting position, the underneath ankle will apply a degree of resistance to the affected leg (this resistance will help to strengthen the knee).

Repeat 5 times.

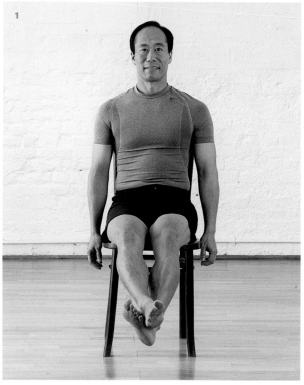

1

For exercises on pp. 213–16

■ Keep your actions gentle, controlled and within your comfort zone.

■ Whether seated or lying, try to not to disturb your pelvis and spine; stay lengthened.

■ If seated, keep your weight evenly distributed.

FURTHER INFORMATION

Further Reading
■ *Return to Life through Contrology* – Joseph Pilates (1945)
■ *Your Health* – Joseph Pilates (1934)
■ *The Pilates Bible* – Lynne Robinson, Lisa Bradshaw and Nathan Gardner (2009)
■ *You're Looking Very Well: The Surprising Nature of Getting Old* – Lewis Wolpert (2011)
■ *Strong Women, Strong Bones* – Miriam E. Nelson (2000)
■ *Training the Over-50s* – Sue Griffin (2006)
■ *Natural Solutions to Menopause* – Marilyn Glenville (2011)
■ *Handbook of the Biology of Ageing* – ed Edward J. Masoro and Steven N. Austad (2001)
■ *The Complete Guide to Teaching Exercise to Special Populations* – Morc Coulson (2011)

Further Information
Advice on health and conditions:
■ www.nhs.uk/Conditions
■ entuk.org
■ www.movementdisorders.org
■ www.mult-sclerosis.org
■ www.macmillan.org.uk/cancerinformation/livingwithandaftercancer/physicalactivity

Advice on healthy eating for older adults:
■ www.nhs.uk/Livewell/over60s/Pages/Nutritionover60.aspx
■ www.ageuk.org.uk/health-wellbeing/healthy-eating-landing/
■ www.nia.nih.gov/health/publication/healthy-eating-after-50

Body Control Pilates
For information on Body Control Pilates, including a list of certified teachers, UK and international teacher training courses, workshops, details on public classes at our London centre in Bloomsbury, plus books, DVDs and Pilates equipment, please visit: www.bodycontrolpilates.com

Useful websites
Age Concern and Help the Aged are now Age UK and provide information and advice for older people about benefits, care, age discrimination and computer courses: www.ageuk.org.uk

You can find information on any of the medical conditions mentioned in this book by visiting the following websites: www.nhs.uk

■ **Alzheimer's and Dementia:** www.alzheimers.org.uk; www.nhs.uk/conditions/dementia-guide
■ **Arthritis:** osteoarthritis – www.arthritiscare.org.uk ; rheumatoid arthritis – www.nras.org.uk
■ **Back health:** www.backcare.org.uk
■ **Breast cancer:** www.macmillan.org.uk/Cancerinformation/Livingwithandaftercancer/Physicalactivity/Physicalactivity.aspx; www.breastcancercare.org.uk
■ **Cancer:** www.nacer.org.uk
■ **Diabetes** www.diabetes.org.uk
■ **Eye health:** http://www.eyecaretrust.org.uk/
■ **Heart health:** www.bhf.org.uk
■ **Hip replacements:** www.nhs.uk/conditions/hip-replacement/Pages/Introduction.aspx
■ **Knee replacements:** www.nhs.uk/conditions/knee-replacement/Pages/Kneereplacementexplained.aspx
■ **Mental health:** www.mind.org.uk
■ **Multiple sclerosis:** www.mssociety.org.uk
■ **Osteoporosis:** www.nos.org.uk
■ **Parkinson's:** www.parkinsons.org.uk
■ **Stroke:** www.stroke.org.uk
■ **Women and men's health:** Association of Chartered Physiotherapists in Women's Health – www.acpwh.org.uk

ACKNOWLEDGEMENTS

LYNNE

We didn't cheat! It is hard to believe, but every one of the models in this book is over the age of 40. I'm sure you will agree with me that they look stunning. We cannot thank them enough for their patience as we asked them to 'hold' the exercise positions for the camera (no mean task). They are all superstars. In no particular order: Victor Robinson (I am proud to say that this handsome young man is my father-in-law), Peter Hawke (Jenny's lovely husband), Derrick Chow, Phillip Adams, Body Control Pilates teachers Denyse Weiser, Heidi Monsen, Tracey Davis, Assil Alsaed, Frances Wilkinson, Suzanne Wooder and Body Control Pilates student (hopefully by now teacher!) Andy Roberts. Thank you all.

I had been mulling over the idea of writing a book for older adults for years, but the approach of my 60th birthday in June 2014 gave me the final nudge to get it done. And I couldn't have found a better co-author than the inspiring Carmela Trappa. For the last five years, Carmela has been kind (and brave) enough to be my Pilates teacher – long suffering and patient, she has put me through my paces, wielding a rod of iron. I am now stronger and fitter than I have ever been. I cannot thank you enough, Carmela, for your guidance, wisdom and friendship.

For our medical consultant I needed to look no further than the fabulous Jenny Hawke, who has been teaching Body Control Pilates for over 14 years as well as being a course tutor and physiotherapist. You cannot put a price on her years of experience. Jenny, thank you so much not only for agreeing to help us with the book, but also for your continued support over the last 15 years. You are just fabulous.

Thank you Karen Robb PhD BSc PGCAP MCSP for helping with the breast cancer chapter in this book. We needed a specialist and as Co Chair of the Macmillan Exercise Advisory Group, a member of the Macmillan Cancer Advisory Board, and a Body Control Pilates student/teacher, you were unbelievably generous in stepping up to the job.

As always, my deepest gratitude to my agent Michael Alcock for all his hard work on our behalf! Then I must express my deepest gratitude to Kyle Cathie, our publisher, for giving us the opportunity to write yet another book. Thank you so much for believing in Pilates.

Catharine and Tara, you managed to edit our unwieldy manuscript into a fantastic book. Thank you so much for your patience. Dan (and Alex) your photographs are, as always, beautiful. Marie, your make up took years off us all...

Linda and Richard, thank you for your support and for brightening up my weekday mornings!

These days, I seem to be busier than ever, teacher training in the UK and all over the world. None of this would have been possible without the hard work and creativity of the Body Control Pilates education team and our tutors, who are talented beyond measure. I thank each and every one of you. Then there are the people behind the scenes at our HQ who work tirelessly to make sure that each student and teacher feels part of the ever-growing community. I am unbelievably proud of the work that they all do.

And last I must thank my family. Leigh, Rebecca and Sean, Emily, all the Robinsons (and Bargerons) and the Bakers, I love you all. So will this be the last book? We will see... I feel there's still so much work to be done!

CARMELA

The development of this idea could not be possible without the constant effort of Lynne, Leigh and Rebecca in 'empowering others for greatness'. I owe my deepest gratitude to Lynne for giving the opportunity to be a part of this 'magnus opus' and for her trust professionally and personally. Jenny, I am heartily thankful for sharing your great expertise and your invaluable encouragement and friendship. I wish to thank you both for inspiring me. A special note goes to my beloved Parents and Family: you always enlighten the right paths and support me; thank you.

JENNY

I am privileged to have been a part of writing this lovely book, and want to thank Lynne and Leigh for their belief in me, and their continuing support over the years. Body Control Pilates has given me so much, both personally and professionally. Carmela, I am so grateful both for your friendship and the opportunity to work with you. Your knowledge amazes me and I continue to learn from you! And finally, thanks to my lovely husband, Peter, for his support.

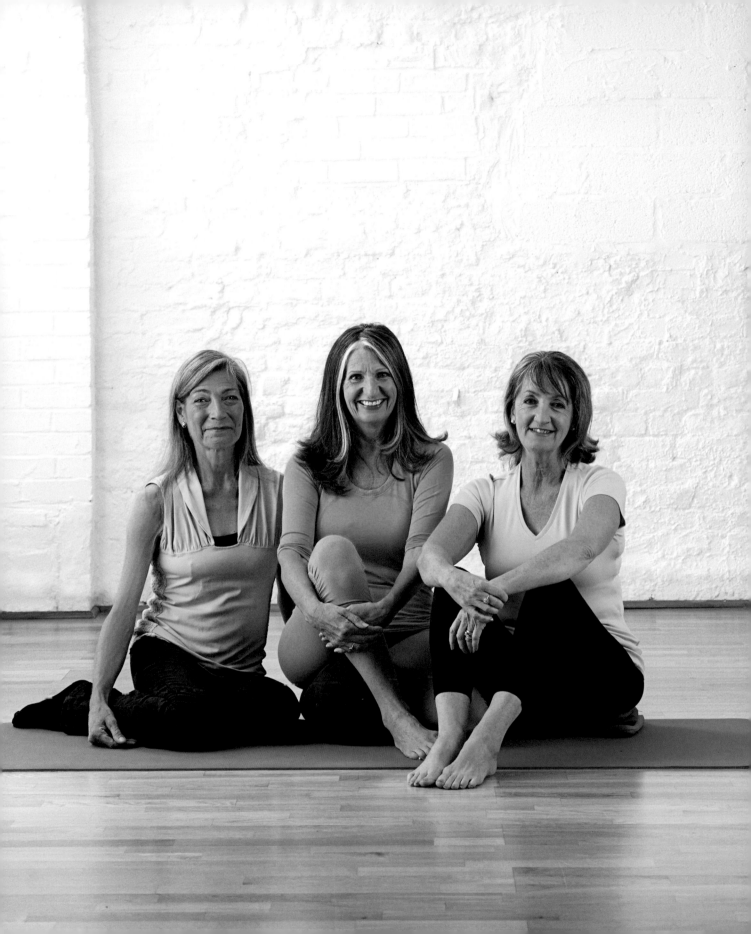

INDEX

'Ageing is not lost youth but a
new stage of opportunity.'
Betty Friedan

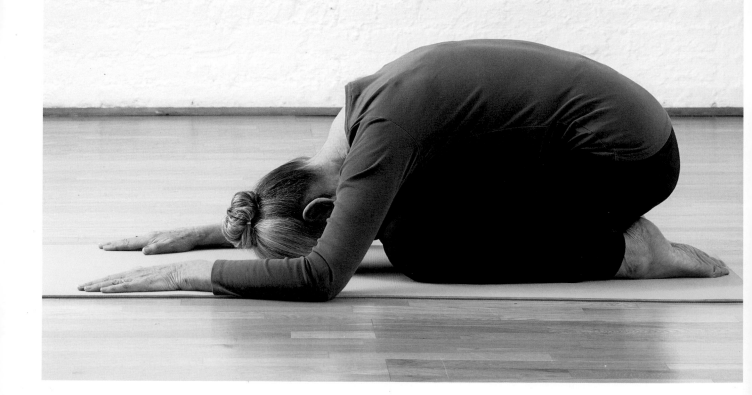